Patient Participation in Health Care Consultations

Patient Participation in Health Care Consultations

Qualitative Perspectives

Edited by Sarah Collins, Nicky Britten, Johanna Ruusuvuori and Andrew Thompson

McGraw Hill
Open University Press

Open University Press
McGraw-Hill Education
McGraw-Hill House
Shoppenhangers Road
Maidenhead
Berkshire
England
SL6 2QL

email: enquiries@openup.co.uk
world wide web: www.openup.co.uk

and Two Penn Plaza, New York, NY 10121-2289, USA

First published 2007

A catalogue record of this book is available from the British Library

ISBN-13: 978 0 335 21964 3 (pb) 978 0 335 21965 0 (hb)
ISBN-10: 0 335 21964 0 (pb) 0 335 21965 9 (hb)

Library of Congress Cataloging-in-Publication Data
CIP data applied for

Typeset by RefineCatch Limited, Bungay, Suffolk
Printed in Poland by OZ Graf. S.A.
www.polskabook.pl

Cover illustration: 'L'Esprit de Deux' by Jean-Claude Gaugy.
Reproduced with kind permission of the Gaugy Gallery, Santa Fe, New Mexico

The McGraw-Hill Companies

Contents

List of contributors

Nicky Britten, Professor of Applied Health Care Research, Institute of Health and Social Care Research, Peninsula Medical School, Universities of Exeter and Plymouth, England.

Carol Bugge, Senior Lecturer, Department of Nursing, University of Stirling, Scotland.

John Chatwin, Research Fellow, School of Healthcare Studies, University of Leeds, England.

Sarah Collins, Lecturer in Health Care Communication, Department of Health Sciences and Hull-York Medical School, University of York, England.

Rowena Field, Homoeopathic Practitioner, York, England.

Joseph Gafaranga, Lecturer, Department of Theoretical and Applied Linguistics, University of Edinburgh, Scotland.

Aled Jones, Lecturer, School of Health Science, University of Wales, Swansea, Wales.

Pirjo Lindfors, Assistant Professor of Health Science, School of Public Health, University of Tampere, Finland.

Anssi Peräkylä, Professor of Sociology, Department of Sociology, University of Helsinki, Finland.

Johanna Ruusuvuori, Assistant Professor in Social Psychology, Department of Sociology and Social Psychology, University of Tampere, Finland.

Fiona Stevenson, Lecturer in Medical Sociology, Department of Primary Care and Population Sciences, Royal Free and University College, London Medical School, England.

Andrew Thompson, Senior Lecturer in Advanced Quantitative Methods, School of Social and Political Studies, University of Edinburgh, Scotland.

Ian Watt, Professor of Primary and Community Care, Department of Health Sciences, University of York, England.

List of illustrations

Figures

Tables

Foreword

Communicating with and involving patients

Helen Lawal and Sue Lawal

In our roles as health care professionals (we are a medical student and a nurse practitioner), we believe that patient participation, and how it can be facilitated through communication, are of paramount importance. This book provides an invaluable source of ideas for reflecting on our practice, and for learning more about patient participation.

To introduce what we regard as the central themes in this book, we present, from our conversation, our views on communication and patient involvement in health care consultations.

Why is communication important in health care?

HL: As a medical student starting out, I tended not to think about communication as part of the learning process. It was not until I began to encounter difficulties communicating with patients (which came in abundance in my first clinical encounters!) that I realized just how important it is. Having the clinical scientific knowledge is nothing, if you don't have the ability to communicate effectively. I see the communication skills I have acquired as life skills which I can apply to many social situations, whereas the scientific knowledge I have gained is only applicable in one context.

SL: As a junior nurse, I acquired communication skills from helping patients with very personal, intimate activities of daily living. I was also required to reassure, comfort and support patients through examinations, diagnostic techniques and treatments being carried out by doctors. As a result, I learned to communicate with the patient on a very different level to that of my medical colleagues. I feel that nursing consultations are often characterized by a closeness and mutuality which patients find comforting. Most of the patients I see have a chronic condition that cannot be cured, only managed. Such conditions can cause a sense of loss and heightened vulnerability.

Why and how do patients want to be involved?

HL: As a student, my encounters with patients thus far have been different to those I will experience later on in my journey as a qualified doctor. The patients whom I have met on placement have volunteered their time, they are keen to be involved and are obviously aware that they are seeing a student, not a qualified professional, therefore the dynamics of such interactions are not realistic. As a student you sometimes come across the 'expert patient' who seems to know everything about their condition, more than you feel you will ever know (!) and who is expert in being questioned by students. It does seem, though, that most patients are quite happy to talk about themselves, providing the questions are appropriate and the professional shows empathy and genuine interest.

SL: I have met very few people who do not want to be actively involved in their care decisions. The degree of involvement does vary, however, and one has to assess where the patient wants the health professional to be at any one time on a continuum ranging from paternalism to autonomy.

How do we – or can we – try to involve people in consultations?

HL: It is often said that a patient tells you their diagnosis, if you listen carefully enough. At my medical school there is a strong emphasis on the use of active listening, silences and patient empowerment as an integral part of consultations. These are techniques which, when used successfully, allow the patient to tell their story, thus addressing the patient's agenda, and not just the health professional's. I have learnt that involving patients is about confidence in using certain skills and techniques, for example, allowing silences, and feeling comfortable with yourself, consequently making the patient feel at ease. Though this is something that comes with experience, I appreciate that even very experienced professionals (like my mum) are still learning.

SL: I like to think of the patient and myself as partners in care. I have the clinical knowledge but they are the ones actually experiencing the condition and I encourage them to share their experiences, so that I can tailor my clinical advice and approach to their individual needs. Having said that, no consultation can be entirely patient-led, as in the real world there are time constraints which require you to keep the subject matter under control! With chronic conditions, each consultation is part of a journey, one that may continue over months or years. Over time, a relationship builds between my patient and myself; a relationship which I like to regard as a partnership in care. Such partnerships can be immensely rewarding for both parties.

Preface

The contributors to this book first met in 2001 when patient participation and partnership were high on the policy and research agenda, shortly after the publication of the *NHS Plan*. Then, we began a series of seminars on the theme of patient participation in health care consultations. The series brought together over 100 people from a variety of lay, professional and academic backgrounds, from across the UK and some from Finland and the USA. Through those interdisciplinary meetings, the ideas presented in this book were developed.

The seminar series and the writing of this book have been, rather like the topic they study, a collaborative project; one that thrives on participation. Our seminar discussions, for example, were led by a variety of speakers who reflected different, often highly diverse, approaches. This allowed us to consider the practicalities and limitations of different health care settings. But it also allowed us to point out to one another creativity in a situation which, to the speaker, in their everyday work, was apparently routine.

As one health professional wrote, after listening to a patient talk:

> The lasting impression for me is Bev's deferential reaction to being asked to speak. When she introduced herself, she professed to feeling somewhat 'out of her depth' in front of the audience. In fact, the very opposite was true as I was left feeling out of my depth after her account of her experiences as a patient with health professionals.

In similar ways, we hope that people reading this book will use it to expand their thinking about participation, to consider perspectives other than their own, to reflect on their experience, and to apply these in their own practice – whether in consulting with patients or professionals, in teaching a class of students, or in designing and conducting research on the topic.

Acknowledgements

This book would not have been possible without the thoughtful and lively discussions among the participants in our seminar series, 'Patient participation in health care consultations', funded by the Economic and Social Research Council (reference no. R451265121). Paul Drew, Vikki Entwistle, Ken Gilhooly and Anne Walker were the other core members, and the following people also contributed: Helen Alexander, Steve Ariss, Angela Barnard, Rachel Barnard, Tracey Bennett, Yvonne Birks, Diana Bleeck, Anne Bradshaw, Lynn Calman, Joyce Campbell, Jill Dales, Zelda di Blasi, Louise Duncan, Jon Emery, Bev Emmerson, Rowena Fellingham, Rowena Field, Jackie Goode, G. Goodman, Richard Hails, Neva Haites, F. Hanson, Gwen Harlow, Imren Hassan, Trine Heinemann, John Heritage, Guro Huby, Rosie Illingworth, Moira Kelly, Celia Kitzinger, Sue Lawal, Fiona Lobban, John Local, Pete Madeley, Margaret Maxwell, Dorothy McCaughan, Jean McKendree, Angela McLelland, Stewart Mercer, Chiara Monzoni, Penny Morris, Audrey Morrison, Andrea Nelson, Sarah Nettleton, Alicia O'Cathain, Susan O'Meara, Delia Orr, Heather Parker, Jill Pattendon, Sarah Peters, Anne Phillips, Pauline Rayner, David Reilly, Penny Rhodes, Joanna Richardson, Helen Roberts, Joy Santon, Bekki Shaw, Zoë Skea, Betty Smith, Judith Smith, Cath Snape, John Spencer, Mike Stone, Vivien Swanson, Julie Thomas, Tony Tolhurst, Jean Turner, Tim Vincent, Alex Walter, Helen Warburton, Pairote Wilainuch, Sue Wilkinson and Tony Wootton.

We would also like to thank: Jonathan Silverman, Stewart Mercer and the other anonymous reviewers of this book; Gill Collins and Lesley Sherwood for so generously hosting our editorial meetings; Jean-Claude and Michelle Gaugy for kind permission to reproduce Jean-Claude Gaugy's painting 'L'Esprit de Deux' on the front cover of our book; Susan Margitts, Joan Smith and Jessica Collins for their invaluable secretarial help; the staff at Open University Press, particularly Rachel Gear and Rachel Crookes, for their support during the production of this book; Susan Dunsmore for her careful copy-editing; Sue Lawal (nurse practitioner) and Helen Lawal (medical student), mother and daughter respectively, for writing the Foreword to this book. The Afterword was written by someone who is a health care assistant, student nurse, parent and patient. She wishes to remain anonymous; but we thank her for writing the final words that highlight the importance of considering patient participation from different personal perspectives.

PART I

Setting the Scene: Debates on Patient Participation and Methods for Studying it

1 Understanding the process of patient participation

Sarah Collins, Nicky Britten, Johanna Ruusuvuori and Andrew Thompson

Commentary

A number of trends, pressures and policy shifts are promoting greater patient involvement in health care delivery through consultations, treatments and continuing care. However, while the literature on different methods of involvement is growing fast, little attention has been given so far to the role which patients themselves wish to play, or to the conceptual meanings behind involvement or participation.

This introductory chapter sets the scene for the book by delineating areas of research relating to patient participation in health care consultations. It outlines some findings from previous research, models for practice that reflect aspects of patient participation, and some interventions designed to promote it.

Against the background of this existing work, this chapter introduces the potential of qualitative methods and empirical research, the orientation of this book, for understanding what patient participation means, how it works, how it may be practised, and how it may be measured.

> The fact is that food varies, and that is what makes it so interesting. Today's piece of cod may be slightly thicker, has larger or finer flakes or thicker skin, than yesterday's. One brand of butter may be different from another. Olive oil changes with every bottle; that is part of its joy. So how can anyone be so pedantic as to give exact timings? Each egg, each steak, each potato is different and will behave in a different way in the pan. That is what cooking is about, and that is why it is essential to understand what you are doing rather than just mindlessly following a recipe.
>
> (From *Appetite* by Nigel Slater 2000: 34)

Introduction

In recent years, patient participation (and patient involvement and partnership) have gained increasing prominence in health care. Patient participation has been prioritized in policy initiatives, has provided the impetus for research programmes, and has found expression in recommendations for professional practice.

Debates about participation reflect a growing unease with the paternalistic philosophy that has traditionally dominated the view of health care consultation, and within which patients were assumed to play minimal and passive roles. Recent decades have seen a ground shift towards initiatives which encourage health care service users to view themselves as active participants in consultations, with individual rather than homogenized needs, and which encourage health care professionals to provide a service which seeks to achieve this. Calls for increased participation from patients and the public are evident in government policy. For example, in the UK, the Inquiry into the tragedy at the Bristol Royal Infirmary (2001) concluded by advocating greater participation by patients and the public. A series of UK health policy documents (Department of Health 2000; 2001; Scottish Executive Health Department 2000; 2003; National Assembly for Wales 2001) prioritize the 'patients' voice' and patients' active roles in their health care. To quote two examples: 'In the twentieth century NHS patients were assumed to be passive recipients of care. In the twenty-first century NHS patients will be active partners in care' (Department of Health 2001: 23); and 'The patients' voice is recognised as being centrally important in the drive for service improvement. [Patients] want to be cared for by professionals who understand their needs and concerns' (National Assembly for Wales 2001: 34). Statements such as these are paralleled in health policy on an international scale.

There are also NHS initiatives to encourage patient and public involvement in health care planning and delivery. One is the Expert Patients Programme (Department of Health 2001) which recognizes that people with chronic diseases are often experts in their own conditions. Another is the involvement of patients and patient groups in communication training for health care professionals, for example, the Patients Accelerating Change initiative, and the use of simulated patients in consultation skills teaching (Spencer and Dales 2006).

From an academic viewpoint, many researchers have investigated patient participation, or similar phenomena such as patient enablement, involvement or partnership, in the past few decades. They have done so for two main reasons. Some promote patient participation in its own right. In the words of Guadagnoli and Ward (1998: 337), 'patient participation in decision making is justified on humane grounds alone and is in line with a patient's right to self-determination'. Others advocate patient participation on the grounds that it will lead to benefits such as improved patient satisfaction, co-operation with health professionals, better management of disease, increased trust and enhanced patient–professional relationships. For example, Coulter (2002) argues that involving patients in treatment and management decisions improves the appropriateness, safety and outcome of care, while at the same time reducing the number of complaints and risk of litigation.

How are these ideals and standards to be realized in practice? A number of obstacles stand in the way of their achievement. One is that, in practice, achieving patients' involvement in their care presents difficulties. Health professionals are increasingly encouraged to deliver patient-centred care, to communicate with their patients and to promote patient participation in consultations but the evidence suggests that patient-centred care and shared decision-making are not widely practised, that many health professionals lack the requisite skills and guidance, and that the contexts in which health care is delivered (including socio-economic influences, work pressures and resource limitations) bring their own constraints. The majority of patient complaints to disciplinary bodies relate to the breakdown of communication between patients and doctors (BMA Board of Medical Education 2004). The literature on shared decision-making has shown that practitioners do not involve patients to any great extent (Stevenson et al. 2000; Elwyn et al. 2005; Ford et al. 2006). Low rates of competency in involving patients in decisions have been detected in formal assessments of doctors' consultation skills (Campion et al. 2002). Similarly, in nursing, despite its long-standing association with the ideals of patient participation and individualized care, there has been little evidence of their application in practice (Cahill 1996; Hartrick 1997).

These difficulties in achieving patient participation are compounded by the increasing diversity in areas of health care, and the increasing variability in patients' expectations. Patients have greater access to information about diagnosis, treatment and care, and are becoming more actively involved, for example, by bringing their choices about treatment to consultations (Richards 1998; Department of Health 2001). At the same time, there continue to be limits to, and uniqueness in, individuals' experiences of health care, for while some patients expect greater understanding and involvement, others want little (for example, Sutherland et al. 1989; Street 1991; Little et al. 2001; Barratt 2005).

Such developments present real communication challenges for health professionals and patients. They demand high levels of sensitivity and flexibility on the part of the health professional in managing the consultation, establishing shared understanding, and accommodating patient and biomedical perspectives. The onus on health professionals to adapt their communication approach to meet individual patients' needs is reiterated in many professional, policy and research documents (for example, Charles et al. 1999; Department of Health 2001; Elwyn et al. 2001; General Medical Council 2001; Stewart 2001; Fallowfield et al. 2002; Coulter and Magee 2003; Hasman et al. 2006).

A related and perhaps more fundamental source of difficulties concerns the fact that, despite the many studies of patient participation, there is little consensus about what participation means. While it may be relatively easy to prescribe or advocate participation (whether in a research project, in a policy document, or in a clinic), it is less easy to understand how it works, or how to make it happen. Practising and facilitating participation between people require skill, understanding, and competence: something more (to borrow Nigel Slater's words above) than 'mindlessly following a recipe'.

In approaching the study and practice of patient participation, this book views communication in the health care consultation as a central influence. The consultation is a principal arena in which patient participation is enacted, may be encouraged and also restricted. Through the consultation, activities such as information exchange, decision-making about treatment, symptom description, and so on, are played out; and how they are played out depends in a large part on communication.

This book sets out to explore the meaning and the practice of patient participation – what participation means, how it works and how it may be promoted. By taking the consultation as the focal point of investigation, this book recognizes the central part played by communication. This is not to deny the importance of the wider context (see Entwistle and Watt 2006), aspects of which are invariably referenced and mirrored in any single patient–health professional encounter. Rather, it is argued here, processes of interaction in the consultation can provide the site of study for that wider context. In each chapter in this book, the consultation is the common reference point for those who contributed (as citizen, health professional or patient) and for the views they expressed. This book is about communication, but it is also about using communication as a way of understanding various influences on the process of participation, many of which extend outside an individual health care encounter.

In pursuit of an understanding of what patient participation means, the next section provides a review of recent developments in health care research and practice that have prioritized patient participation and sought to define it. Building on this background, the third section proposes a more inclusive view of, and approach to the study of, patient participation. The contributions of this book are then outlined. In the concluding section, readers are invited to take different routes through the book, depending on their particular interests and motivations in the study and practice of patient participation.

Previous research on patient participation in health care consultations

Patient participation is not a new concept. It needs to be understood within the context of long-standing debates about the doctor–patient relationship (Balint 1957), the development of an approach to the consultation that integrates the biomedical and health professional agenda with the patients' concerns and expectations (McWhinney 1972); a tradition of observational research that pays attention to what actually happens in consultations (Davis 1978; Strong 1979); and Tuckett et al.'s (1985) groundbreaking work demonstrating that patients and doctors do not share or exchange ideas to a great degree.

The past decade has witnessed a wealth of research literature and associated interventions for professional practice which make explicit reference to patient participation. The review presented here is necessarily selective, and the divisions it makes are somewhat artificial; the fields presented separately here overlap in practice and share some similar concerns. For other reviews and useful summaries of research relating to patient participation, see Chapter 3 in this volume; Cahill (1996); Robinson (2003); Farrell (2004); and Heritage and Maynard (2006).

In order to introduce the particular strengths of this book, this review of previous research is organized according to the various approaches that have been taken to studying patient participation. Quantitative studies have tended to focus on measuring concepts such as information exchange, shared decision-making, patient enablement, verbal dominance and communication control. They have also developed conceptual models and interventions to promote forms of patient participation and their observed effects. Qualitative studies have tended to focus on professional responsibility and behaviour, and on details of observed and recorded communication in consultations, as well as on the structure of the consultation and its phases.

Quantitative approaches

A number of coding systems have been developed to study patients' participation and associated topics such as shared decision-making in consultations. Some of these systems have their origins in the social psychological Interaction Process Analysis (IPA) system developed in the 1950s (Bales 1951). Others have developed as a consequence of attempts to measure the distribution and determinants of quality of care (Howie et al. 2004). These approaches have provided useful information on, for example, the extent to which patients talk in the consultation, and factors influencing the interpersonal effectiveness of the health professional, such as length of consultation or continuity of care.

Roter's Interactional Analysis Scale (RIAS) is one of the most influential of these coding systems (Roter and Larson 2002). Roter (2000) used the term relationship-centred care to connote the optimal form of patient–physician relationship. She characterized this as medically functional, informative, facilitative, responsive and participatory. In describing participatory relationships, she claimed that physicians have an obligation to help patients assume an authentic and responsible role in the medical dialogue and in decision-making. In order to measure relationship-centred care, she devised two quantitative indicators: verbal dominance and communication control. These indicators were used to analyse a large corpus of primary care consultations which Roter described as either biomedical or participatory. The biomedical exchanges accounted for two-thirds of the consultations. The participatory consultations were those in which the physicians were less verbally dominant and patients had more communication control. In these consultations, there was more talk in the psychosocial domain, with the exception of consumerist consultations during which physicians provided patients with much biomedical information.

Models of the consultation

Models of patient-centred consultations and shared decision-making reflect a similar orientation towards physician behaviour, and are widely employed in the teaching and training of health professionals. The patient-centred process, long advocated by Stewart et al. (1995), has six interactive components. These are: (1) exploring both the disease and the illness experience; (2) understanding the whole person; (3) finding common ground; (4) incorporating prevention and health promotion; (5) enhancing the patient–doctor relationship; and (6) being realistic. The Calgary–Cambridge guide to the medical consultation, which is widely used in doctors' training, identifies tasks under five headings: (1) initiating the session; (2) gathering information; (3) physical examination; (4) explanation and planning; and (5) closing the session (Kurtz et al. 1998). Similarly, Elwyn et al. (2003a) set out nine professional competences for shared decision-making. These are: (1) problem definition; (2) portrayal of equipoise; (3) portrayal of options; (4) checking the patient's understanding; (5) exploring the patient's ideas, concerns and expectations; (6) establishing the patient's role preference; (7) decision-making; (8) deferment if necessary; and (9) making arrangements to review the decision if appropriate.

Interventions

Researchers have also developed and evaluated interventions to increase patient participation in health care consultations. These interventions have been targeted at different aspects of participation, and have been evaluated using a range of outcome measures (for a recent review, see Haywood et al. 2006).

Middleton et al. (2006), for example, took a dual approach, targeting both patient and professional behaviours. They ran workshops for general practitioners to increase their awareness of patients' agendas. They then provided the patients of these doctors with agenda forms for the patients to complete in the waiting room before their consultations. Patients were encouraged to write down their concerns and show them to their doctor. The results of this randomized controlled trial showed a small increase in the number of problems identified and a commensurate increase in consultation length. The patients were more satisfied with the consultations, but there was no change in the number of 'by the way' presentations of extra problems, arising after the doctor considered the consultation to be finished.

Another much-cited study (Greenfield et al. 1985) used an intervention in which patients were helped to read their medical records before the consultation, and were trained to ask questions and negotiate medical decisions. Assistants coached patients to write down any questions that they found potentially embarrassing. Results showed that patients who received the intervention were more satisfied afterwards and reported fewer physical limitations than the control group. However, despite the overt encouragement, patients did not ask significantly more questions but instead found indirect methods for obtaining more information from their physicians.

Mercer and Howie (2006) employed a measure of consultation quality (CQI-2), using questionnaire techniques, to explore the interpersonal effectiveness of general practitioners. This measure was devised to capture elements of consultation 'outcome' (patient enablement), 'process' (continuity of care), and 'structure' (consultation length), which were recorded for each participating patient's consultation. Patients were also asked about their confidence in their GP, whether they felt able to discuss problems with their GP, whether they would recommend their doctor to others, and about their overall satisfaction with the consultation. Doctors completed the same empathy measure, and were also asked to rate their general performance and their view of the importance of empathy in consultations. The results revealed, among other findings, positive correlations between doctors' CQI-2 scores and their view of ideal consultation length; that doctors who felt patients didn't value the job they did had lower CQI-2 scores; and highly significant correlations between CQI-2 scores and mean patient scores for confidence in the doctor, whether they would recommend the doctor to others, and their overall satisfaction. This application of the CQI-2 measure suggests some significant links between empathy, enablement, consultation length, and a doctor's interpersonal effectiveness.

These studies and others have shown that it is possible to increase patient participation from a low base level, although at present it remains unclear how transferable these interventions are to routine clinical practice.

The problem with these quantitative coding systems, questionnaires, and models of the consultation is that they do not tell us how the coded actions relate to one another, for example, how the patients' information-seeking actions are interpreted by the health professionals, and whether or not such actions on the part of the patient receive a response; or how the length of a consultation might influence the way in which topics are talked about and whether and how an individual patient's priorities and concerns are characterized and addressed. They have not examined the interaction, the specific ways in which the talk of one participant influences that of the other, nor considered the context in which the interaction takes place. Thus, they do not provide insights into how the actual interaction enables the development of rapport, for example, or into the details of how a health professional behaviour, such as interpersonal effectiveness, is actually enacted and practised through communication in the consultation. Their findings, however, do point to the normative structure of medical consultations, and suggest that a more nuanced approach to understanding patient participation is necessary.

Qualitative approaches

Another area of work on patient participation concerns qualitative analyses of communication between patients and health professionals. One of the strengths of much of this research is that it has not specifically set out to study patient participation, and therefore reveals particular facets of it. A range of studies seek to show how the interrelationship between the patient's concerns and the biomedical agenda is a dynamic, constantly at play in the consultation. They demonstrate the co-presence of patient and doctor perspectives, the different competencies that the patient and the doctor each bring, and the interactive consulting processes through which the agenda is constructed.

In its recognition of different voices in the consultation, Mishler's (1984) work has been particularly influential. Mishler distinguished two 'voices' – the voice of the lifeworld that represents the natural attitude of everyday life and the voice of medicine that represents the technical-scientific assumptions of medicine. In his analyses, Mishler began by noting the dominant voice of medicine. He provided examples of how patients' meanings conveyed in the voice of the lifeworld tended to be treated by doctors as non-medically relevant.

Mishler's work was motivated by a concern to isolate features of discourse that, in a medical encounter, might 'retrieve the possibilities of a more humane medical interview' (1984: 139); and he identified qualities of interaction that have since been substantiated in the work of others. These qualities, he observed, differ according to whether the doctor integrates the two voices, or proceeds in the voice of medicine alone, and ignores the voice of the lifeworld.

A related theme concerns the patient's and doctor's discrepant competencies. While doctors are communicatively competent in both voices, most patients are communicatively competent only in the voice of the lifeworld. To the patient, the doctor's questions come one after another with no apparent connection between them, and do not enable the patient to maintain the flow of his/her story. The doctor must translate the patient's lifeworld statements into medical terms, and medical statements of problems into patients' terms.

Mishler's work pointed to two significant dimensions of consultations. One concerned the two voices, their characteristics, and where and how each was used. The other concerned the different competencies of the patient and the doctor. These dimensions are reflected in the work of Barry et al. (2001).

Barry et al. applied Mishler's conceptualization of the two voices to their analyses of data which included interviews with patients and doctors, and a measure of consultation outcomes, as well as recordings of the consultations themselves.

The four patterns of communication that Barry et al. (2001) identified reveal a more complex interrelation between the two voices than Mishler (1984) previously showed. 'Strictly Medicine' described those encounters in which both doctor and patient used the voice of medicine exclusively. This pattern was found in consultations for acute problems, and it appeared that these consultations were most effective. However, in some cases the pattern resulted in major misunderstandings on diagnosis and prescription. In 'Lifeworld Blocked' consultations, glimpses of the lifeworld revealed the patients' concerns, but these were not taken up by the doctor and were blocked by the voice of medicine. In 'Lifeworld Ignored', only the patients used the voice of the lifeworld, while the doctors conducted the whole of their communication in the voice of medicine. In the final group, the Mutual Lifeworld, both doctors and patients predominantly used the voice of the lifeworld. The authors describe (Barry et al. 2001: 496): 'a much more relaxed feel to these consultations, with more evidence of responsiveness on the part of the doctors in recognising and respecting the patient's unique situation'.

They accounted for this in part through the psychological nature of the patients' presenting problems, the sources of which belonged more in the lifeworld. The greatest dissonance was found in consultations about chronic physical problems. To the patients, these conditions were a lifeworld issue, though the doctors seemed to regard them as a physical issue requiring the voice of medicine (Barry et al. 2001: 504).

These two studies (Mishler 1984; Barry et al. 2001) demonstrate ways in which the consultation agenda is defined interactionally. Through the interaction, patients' concerns and biomedical perspectives are shaped and are accorded their respective place. These studies illuminate the patient's part in the process; and they show that there are choices or alternatives open to both patient and professional in the interaction, in particular, ways in which the doctor's reasoning processes, and the sources of coherence which underlie the consultation management, can be made more transparent for the patients.

In these respects, the studies supply insight into what is at stake in constructing the consultation agenda, what gains recognition and import, and the problems in understanding that arise between the patient and the health professional. But their descriptions of the communication – e.g. 'open' and 'closed' questions (Mishler 1984), the 'relaxed feel' and 'doctors' responsiveness' in Mutual Lifeworld consultations (Barry et al. 2001) – leave a great deal unsaid.

To uncover the intricacies of the sequential organization and delivery of communication, and to determine the specific consequences for patients' participation, research in the field of conversation analysis can be helpful. While conversation analysis is not the only way of analysing interaction in consultations, it does provide a detailed and well-established method of understanding social interaction and the processes through which participation is realized. In this book, we have employed conversation analysis as our main approach to describing and understanding forms of patient participation in consultations. We have done so as a means of drawing on data that allows us to observe what actually happens, and to investigate what patient participation actually means and what it looks like in practice. Thus, we are using conversation analysis, along with other methods, to illuminate observable forms of patient participation; and we do not wish to imply that conversation analysis is the only method.

In conversation analysis (hereafter CA), the consultation is viewed as realized by health professionals and patients in and through the interaction that takes place between them. The participants present and acknowledge concerns, ask and answer questions, give and accept or reject treatment proposals. Consequent turns of talk by the participants form sequences of action, which in turn build up into phases of activities that can be seen to comprise the main 'task' of the consultation, and, on the societal level, the purpose of the institution. In doctor–patient consultations, the main task and its purpose are to attend to, and find treatment for, the patient's health-related problems; while in hospital admission interviews carried out by nurses, it might be to record general information about the patient, in relation to their medical history and their activities of daily living. In CA research, the consultation is regarded as consisting of phases of activities that have been located in empirical research based on video or audio recordings of actual consultations. The phases observed in doctor–patient consultations are the opening of the consultation, the problem presentation, verbal examination (including history-taking), physical examination, discussions of treatment, and closing (see also Byrne and Long 1976). Depending on the nature of the consultation (whether it is a first consultation or a follow-up, an acute and visible concern or a chronic one) as well as on other contingencies that may occur in consultations, some phases may be left out or they may occur in various orders, and/or overlapping each other.

Particular features of the opening lines of the consultation have been shown to shape the expression of the patient's concerns (Coupland et al. 1992; Ruusuvuori 2000; Gafaranga and Britten 2003; Heritage and Robinson 2006a; Robinson 2006). For example, Ruusuvuori (2000) analysed the opening phase of primary care consultations to consider how control is managed in interaction. She identified the patient's use of a narrative format to regulate the space for describing the 'reason for visit', and observed that the patient could take 'temporary control' through an extended turn, part of which involved justifying the reason for visiting. The doctor, in response, tended to negotiate the move away from the patient's presenting concern in such a way as to also acknowledge its import. To give another example, Robinson (2006) depicts the different designs of doctors' questions for eliciting patients' concerns, with each design reflecting an orientation to a particular type of problem – new, follow-up, and routine re-check. Patients, in response, demonstrate their understanding of the shaping role these questions play in characterizing their problems; and they may resist answering if the question does not reflect the nature of their presenting problem.

While the problem presentation is described as the prime opportunity for a patient to voice concerns (Heritage and Robinson 2006a), the history-taking phase which follows it has repeatedly been shown to be a relatively restricted environment for patient-initiated actions (Stivers and Heritage 2001: 165; and see Heath 1992; Robinson 2003; Gill and Maynard 2006). Boyd and Heritage (2006) and Stivers and Heritage (2001) observe a variety of resources by means of which, in the course of history-taking, patients can resist question agendas and expand beyond them. Gill and Maynard's (2006) study of patients' explanations for their illnesses highlights the dilemmas faced by patients and doctors in offering and receiving explanations. Patients try to offer explanations in a relevant sequential environment (the history-taking) while not disrupting this information-gathering phase, and doctors can then find themselves in the position of receiving and acknowledging patients' explanations prior to having gathered all the data necessary for analysis.

Moving on from history-taking to the other aspect of information-gathering, the physical examination phase, Heritage and Stivers (1999) show how the on-line commentary that physicians provide can serve both to provide reassurance for the patient, and to justify and forecast an upcoming diagnostic evaluation. This on-line commentary is demonstrated, in many cases, to shape patients' expectations towards a certain outcome – a no-problem evaluation.

In terms of diagnosis and treatment decisions, Heritage and Maynard's (2006) review of the conversation analysis literature notes less opportunity to participate in diagnosis than in the treatment phase. In the diagnostic phase of the consultation, Peräkylä (1997; 2002) identifies two alternative formats by which doctors deliver diagnoses, one which allows patients to participate in the diagnosis (perhaps by enhancing or resisting it), and another which does not. In discussions about treatment, Stivers (2002) demonstrates how the particulars of the turn design format employed by doctors can engender patients' participation in treatment decisions.

With regard to the closing phase of the consultation, West's (2006) analyses of primary care consultations show that although doctors conduct consultations under certain time pressures, the manner in which they bring them to a close serves to maintain their attentiveness to their patients' interests and thus works to ensure continuity of care and to maintain the doctor–patient relationship.

The conversation analysis studies described above show how patients' concerns are expressed in numerous ways at different points in consultations. This research displays the sensitivities and dilemmas faced by both doctors and patients in their communication of the consultation agenda, and it demonstrates the particular capacity of conversation analysis to handle the intricacies of communication in consultations, as a route to understanding patient participation.

However, the CA research, referenced above, also houses certain biases that may stand in the way of achieving some balanced consideration of exactly what patients and health professionals contribute to the construction and management of the consultation agenda. For the most part, these biases result from the predominant focus of this research on areas such as primary care and doctors' consultations, and on activities such as diagnosis and treatment discussion. Conversation analysts have themselves recognized these preoccupations, and have begun to investigate patient-initiated actions, occasions where patients initiate radical departures from the medical agenda, and patients' hidden agendas and points of view (for example, Drew 2001; Gill and Maynard 2006). However, as CA studies concentrate on analysing the *process* of interaction, they cannot adequately deal with other equally relevant dimensions of the process of patient participation, such as what is left unsaid in the consultation. For those other dimensions, other forms of data, such as patient questionnaires, semi-structured interviews and focus groups are more useful.

Summary

Broadly speaking, the research reviewed in this section can be separated into two strands. One strand has tended to focus on information exchange, shared decision-making, and professional behaviour, and has examined statistical links between their measures and outcome measures such as compliance with medication, professional behaviour, or features of the consultation. It has developed typologies, for example, of the doctor–patient relationship, of shared decision-making, which are often theoretical conceptualizations. The other strand has examined the details of interaction in consultations, and the structures of communication with regard to the consultation's phases. Taken together, these studies outline what might be considered to be essential features of, or prerequisites for, participation.

The studies reported above make important contributions to understanding patient participation but they also display certain limitations. These studies have tended to stand alone, and to take particular stances towards participation. They begin with a particular ideal or conception of participation; emphasize either content, or process; recommend a wholesale, global application of patient participation; exhibit a preoccupation with measuring patient participation and those professional behaviours which may be considered to promote or restrict it; limit their investigation to doctor–patient interaction (as opposed to the consultations of other health professionals such as nurses); and focus, almost exclusively, on primary care.

In sum, these studies can only show us a partial view of patient participation. In this book, we aim to open up a wider view on the subject, by facilitating dialogue between different qualitative approaches to the study of patient participation, by concentrating on what actually happens in real interactions between patients and health professionals, and by studying the process of patient participation.

Building a more comprehensive view of patient participation

This book aims to add to previous analyses and conceptualizations by approaching the question 'what is patient participation?' as a problem to be posed, both in research and in practice.

This book, like those studies reviewed above, assumes that patient participation is desirable and achievable. But it also proposes that, until we understand what patient participation means, and how it works in different contexts, we should be wary of beginning to promote it. Rather than viewing patient participation as a concept or practice to be sold and adopted wholesale, our aim is to develop a more nuanced understanding of its forms and variations; one founded on empirical data and on the expressed views and observable practices of both patients and health professionals. Understanding participation means becoming attuned to variations between individuals, recognizing and accommodating individual sensitivities and different levels of responsiveness at different moments. Thus, this book models a cautious, context-sensitive and questioning approach to the concept and practice of patient participation. In our view, an openness to what patient participation means, and an acknowledgement of its context-sensitivity and changing forms, are necessary to ensure quality in health care.

This book takes a wide view of patient participation. It aims to describe the various forms that patient participation takes, bringing on board its everyday meanings, and not just the significant errors and policy statements, and the questions of professional performance and imposed standards, as presented in the review above. In relation to interventions in health professional practice, this book takes the view that rather than adopting interventions that focus on professional behaviour and responsibility, or giving advice to health professionals about appropriate responses, a more constructive approach is to sensitize health professionals to the complexities and variations of forms of patient participation, according to different contexts. In order to document this diversity, the studies are descriptive in orientation, and focus on the interactional processes that may foster participation, or perhaps restrict it.

The questions this book raises include the following (and see the Educational Supplement, p. 197). What is patient participation, and how can it be studied? Is patient participation assumed to be a good thing? Or is it being questioned? How may patient participation be described? How may it be measured? In what respects may patient participation be recommended and advocated? How can we facilitate it? Can it be effectively taught?

There are certain questions this book does not deal with. These include questions concerning the development of appropriate measures of participation, and the effects of patient participation on health care outcomes. Rather, this book focuses on what participation is, using a range of qualitative approaches, in order to be able to specify it more clearly. Until this is done, it is not possible to devise quantitative measures for participation, or to assess the effects of participation on health care outcomes. In a sense, then, we are going back to the drawing board, and hope that our work will be useful to those wishing to develop measures of participation or to examine the links to outcomes.

The contributions of this book

The book is divided into three parts, and includes educational supplements and an appendix with CA transcription. The introductory Part I (Chapters 1 and 2) outlines the policy background, the conceptual framework, and the research methodologies employed. Continuing the line of argument presented in this chapter, Chapter 2 ('Methods for studying patient participation', Bugge and Jones) invites experimentation with combinations of methods, researcher interpretations, and health professional and patient perspectives, as a means of achieving greater understanding and insight into the concept of patient participation.

In Part II (Chapters 3 to 8), the empirical part concerned with how participation is enacted in practice and in everyday situations, patient participation is explored by reference to a range of types of data, collected in different health care settings. It opens with two chapters (Chapters 3 and 4) which explore health care users' views of participation. Chapter 3 ('The meaning of patient involvement and participation in health care consultations: A taxonomy', Thompson), examines empirical evidence from a qualitative study of the views and preferences of citizens, patients, and members of voluntary/community groups. The extent to which involvement was desired and sought depended on a variety of factors (e.g. type of illness, personal characteristics and patients' relationships with professionals). Participation was seen to occur when there was reciprocity with professionals through dialogue and shared decision-making. Chapter 4 ('What is a good consultation and what is a bad one?' Stevenson) presents patients' views of 'good' and 'bad' consultations, elicited through interviews immediately following from consultations in general practice. The range of patients' responses reflected several influences on their perceptions of involvement: the personalities of health care providers, the way in which consultations are organized, notions of rights and responsibilities, and issues relating to the structural organization of health care.

Chapters 5, 6, 7 and 8 make up the remainder of the empirical section. These chapters focus primarily on recordings of consultations and analyses of interaction. Each one illuminates aspects of structures of communication in consultations, and demonstrates ways in which features of these structures, and their variations, promote or restrict patients' participation. Chapter 5 ('A feeling of equality', Chatwin et al.) explores qualities of communication with reference to a consultation taking place in an NHS homoeopathic hospital. Through detailed consideration of one instance of a consultation opening, accompanied by extracts from a themed discussion and interviews with health professionals, this chapter discusses environmental influences on consultations, and specifies features of the interaction that appear to promote mutual respect and rapport between the patient and the doctor. Chapter 6 ('Patient participation in formulating and opening sequences', Gafaranga and Britten) takes two communication practices in general practice consultations, openings and formulations, that have been studied elsewhere, and re-examines these practices to consider what each one illuminates about the meaning of patient participation, and how it may be promoted. Chapter 7 ('What is patient participation?', Peräkylä et al.) explores patient participation in three different health care settings in Finland (general practice, homoeopathy and psychoanalysis). This chapter provides a comparative description of patients' comments on practitioners' expert statements, and highlights some distinctive features of patient participation in relation to each of these settings and types of activity. Chapter 8 ('Nursing assessments and other tasks', Jones and Collins) describes the constraints on and opportunities for the raising of patients' concerns, as found in interactions between patients and nurses in three different nursing contexts.

Part III (Chapters 9 and 10) draws together the main findings from the collection of studies to present a conceptual and methodological framework for understanding patient participation, and to develop ideas concerning how it may be recommended, fostered and measured. These chapters build on the multi-faceted definition of participation developed through Chapters 1 to 8, to reflect its context-sensitive properties and its interactive and dynamic forms. Chapter 9 ('Components of participation', Peräkylä and Ruusuvuori) considers the methodological dimensions of research on patient participation, and what these reflect about the practice of participation. Chapter 10 ('An integrative approach to patient participation in consultations', Thompson et al.) summarizes the main arguments and findings from this book into a conceptual overview. This overview integrates the various contributions and takes these through from micro-level studies to the macro-level. Its aim is to explore the potential for mapping these contributions into a holistic framework which will enable those working in patient participation to locate their particular area of research, practice, or experience within it.

The final part of the book is a series of educational supplements, linked to the chapters. Each supplement offers additional data examples, discussion questions, analytic exercises, and prompts for teaching and research, in relation to the themes of each chapter.

Contexts for participation

The context for this book is processes of communication in health care consultations. We have deliberately chosen to examine a range of settings and different types of health care practitioner. This range provides more than a broad basis for our conclusions; it also invites comparison and exchange of communication practices, across different health care contexts. We consider consultations in primary and secondary care, including homoeopathy, general practice, head and neck cancer outpatient clinics, diabetes in primary care, family planning and psychoanalysis. The practitioners are doctors, nurses, homoeopaths and psychoanalysts, and the chapters include material from the United Kingdom and from Finland. The rationale for studying other types of consultation, in addition to orthodox medical consultations, is that these permit a broader analysis of what patient participation is, and of what it might be, given the very different contexts of practice and world-views of their practitioners. Thus, the study of homoeopathic or psychoanalytic consultations gives us different lenses through which to examine medical consultations.

The chapters represent a diversity of experiences across different patient populations, with a rich variety of empirical data gleaned from consultations, interviews, and discussion groups with a range of health service users, patients and professionals. The reader can use the book to make their own comparisons, for example, of the difference between people's stated preferences for involvement and actual consultations (Chapters 4, 5 and 6); between forms of patient participation in conventional medical consultations and forms of patient participation in homoeopathy and psychoanalysis (Chapters 5 and 7); or between nurses' and doctors' communication (Chapters 2 and 8). Our conceptual overview (presented in Chapters 9 and 10) is derived from these diverse sources, ranging from analyses of actual consultations to the views of those not currently in need of health care.

Methods for studying patient participation

As well as examining a range of contexts, this book also uses a range of qualitative methods, as each method on its own can only provide a partial picture. Chapter 2 shows how a combination of methods can provide a more rounded view. As the focus of the book is on the consultation, several chapters are based on recordings of actual consultations, for which we have principally employed conversation analysis (Chapters 2, 5, 6, 7 and 8). We have also used qualitative interviews, focus groups and themed discussions, non-participant observation and retrospective think aloud techniques (and this range is also echoed in the educational supplements). This range of methods means that our analysis is not confined either to what people say they do (in interviews or focus groups, for example) or to what they can be observed to be doing (in recordings of consultations), but embraces both.

The picture of patient participation presented in this book

In policy documents and in the research literature, the concept of participation is often presented as if it were ubiquitous, as if to suggest that it has a single and commonly understood meaning. This is not the case. As shown in Chapter 3, it is closely related to the concepts of 'involvement', 'collaboration' and even 'partnership'. Chapter 3 explores the meanings of the words 'participation' and 'involvement' to citizens and patients, and the ways in which these meanings might differ from those held by professionals and researchers. For some, silence may represent an obvious form of non-participation, while in Chapter 2 we show how a patient's silence may influence the subsequent course of a consultation. Patient participation may be defined in one way when studying consultations, and in another way when talking to patients afterwards. It may mean one thing to a healthy citizen in a focus group, and another to a patient in a head and neck cancer outpatient clinic, and something else again to a nurse, GP, homoeopath or surgeon. Thus, in this book, we aim to examine the concept of patient participation from a wide range of perspectives. We include the views of citizens, as well as patients; professional, lay and academic perspectives; those in secondary and primary care; in health care policy in nursing and in medicine; in Finland and in the UK. In Chapter 9, we identify five key components of patient participation, each with its specific site of empirical manifestation and each with its own specific research method(s). These components may be used as a conceptual model to inform future research. In the last chapter, we link these components to levels of patient participation and examine the contexts of participation.

How to use this book

The structure of the book is designed to help its readers use it in different ways. An editorial commentary opens each chapter in the book, to introduce themes and highlight the direction being taken. By reading the series of commentaries alone, the reader can gain an overview of the whole book. Each chapter concludes with a summary of recommendations. Linked to each chapter is an educational supplement, with ideas and applications for communication skills teaching and for reflecting on clinical practice. The chapters and supplements can be read in different orders, and the reader can start and stop in different places; read only selected parts, or the book as a whole. The Appendix presents the notation for the Conversation Analysis transcripts used in the book.

The book is intended to progress the reader's understanding and knowledge by one or more of the following routes:

- providing the reader with different ways of characterizing patient participation;
- enabling the reader to see and understand differences between patient and professional perspectives;
- encouraging interdisciplinary thinking and debate;
- enlightening understanding about the process of patient participation.

The book is also intended to inspire the reader, in a number of activities, for example:

- identify a theme for a course assignment;
- create a new taught course, using the educational supplements;
- try out new communication techniques in health care practice;
- review current health care policy;

- review organizational features of health care consultations, clinics, or interdisciplinary team management;
- develop strategies for advising and supporting user groups;
- compile a leaflet based on patients' stories;
- set up a piece of research;
- try a new research method.

The data extracts in themselves can be compared with other examples from students' own research and/or areas of professional practice. The information contained in each chapter can be employed to pose and answer questions with applications in research and in professional practice, such as: 'How can we as professionals make the openings to encounters with patients more therapeutic?', or 'What are the various ways in which patients *wish* to be involved in consultations, compared to how they actually *are* involved?'

Different ways of reading the book reflect different ways of being involved and of participating. We hope that you will find it an enjoyable and stimulating experience.

Recommendations: summary

- Patient participation should always be considered in context: it may mean different things when seen from different perspectives.
- In promoting patient participation either in policy or in practices of health care, we should remain open to its context-sensitivity and changing forms.
- In order to understand the process of patient participation, and thus how to influence and develop measures of participation and its effects on health care outcomes, it is necessary to pay close attention to what actually happens in interactions between patients and health professionals.

2 Methods for studying patient participation

Carol Bugge and Aled Jones

Commentary

This chapter begins with an overview of the range of methods employed by the contributors to this book. The substantive body of the chapter is then dedicated to an illustration of how these various qualitative methods (both alone and in combination) can be used to investigate different research questions in relation to patient participation, drawing on examples from our different studies.

The examples show how, by combining qualitative methods and drawing on a variety of informants and perspectives, a greater understanding of the concept of participation can be achieved than by using any one approach alone. Our collective view of consultation, interview and focus group data has led us to see that at any level of detail, and through any number of viewings, a host of interesting observations can be made. Our understandings of patient participation developed through debate about convergent, discordant and unique findings. This approach, we argue, offers a more comprehensive picture of the complexities of patient participation than is otherwise afforded.

Through this chapter, the reader is similarly invited to scrutinize the material and interpretations presented in this book from a number of angles, and to experiment with different perspectives and approaches, whether in their research or in their professional practice.

Introduction

As described in Chapter 1, patient participation is a complex phenomenon and, as yet, there seems to be little consensus about what it is and what is necessary to achieve it. Reaching an understanding of such a complex phenomenon clearly requires methodological ingenuity.

In this chapter, our aim is to consider the usefulness of combining qualitative research methods for the study of this concept, and to investigate the ways in which collecting and comparing diverse types of data can illuminate understanding of a research problem.

Overview of methods represented in this book

The contributors to this book represent different professional (e.g. nursing, medicine) and academic backgrounds (e.g. sociology, psychology) and each had been involved in at least one study of patient participation. In addition, in developing ideas for the different individual chapters and for the combined message of the book, lay members of the public and other academics and health professionals (see the Acknowledgements) have been involved in discussions and have been significant contributors of ideas.

In their individual studies of patient participation, the contributors to this book have used various qualitative methods for data collection and analysis. These methods include:

- *Conversation analysis* (hereafter CA) of audio- or video-recorded consultations. For example, in one study, patient–nurse interactions during ward assessments were audio-recorded and analysed (see this chapter and Chapter 8).
- *Semi-structured qualitative interviews* with patients, health professionals and citizens. For example, interviews were conducted with patients, immediately following a consultation, to explore their experiences of participation in consultations (see Chapter 4).
- *Retrospective 'think aloud' techniques* with patients and health professionals. For example, recordings of consultations were replayed (in part or whole) to prompt patients' and health professionals' reflections on what they were thinking about at specific points in the consultation (see this chapter).
- *Non-participant observation* of interactions and of health care environments. For example, interactions between nurses and patients during ward admissions were observed (see Chapter 8).
- *Focus groups* involving moderators, with patients, health professionals,

members of the general public and of voluntary organizations. For example, discussions about the forms of involvement patients seek in their own health care (see Chapter 3).

Table 2.1 (see pp. 25–6) presents the main methods used in this book. It outlines, in terms of participation, what each method may be most usefully employed to study, what it may be less useful for studying, and the types of research question that the method may usefully address.

For an introduction to these methods and pointers for further reading, see Pope and Mays (2006). The strengths and weaknesses of individual methods are well debated elsewhere and we will therefore not revisit these debates here.

This chapter will now demonstrate the ways in which these different qualitative research methods, presented in the studies in this book, have contributed to the development of our understanding of patient participation.

Mixing methods in the study of patient participation

In health services research, the use of a range of different methods can provide a more rounded view of a complex phenomenon, such as patient participation, than is possible with a single methodological approach. Different methods provide different insights, and in this chapter we show how it is possible to increase the scope of what we know about patient participation in health care consultations by comparing these various insights.

We will focus on examples of individual methods and of combined methods and how they illuminate (or occlude) features of participation in health care consultations. In particular, we consider the added value of using mixed methods to study patient participation in health care consultations.

Applications of methods

Three examples are presented in the following sections which illustrate different ways in which we used our methods within and across studies, and the outcomes of using and combining methods in these ways.

Example 1 Using different methods and researchers in one study

This example is drawn from a single study in which patients and health professionals were interviewed and consultations were video-recorded (Entwistle et al. 2004; Collins et al. 2005; Bugge et al. 2006) and in which researchers from

Table 2.1 Overview of methods for studying participation and their uses

	A more useful method for	*A less useful method for*	*Types of research questions*
Conversation analysis of audio- and video-recorded consultations	• Studying details of interaction between participants in consultations • Objectively looking at the participation that occurs in consultations and in sequences of interaction • Studying what actually happens in consultations	• Considering what is not made visible in the interaction	• What opportunities are made available to participants for taking part in consultations? • In what ways do patients participate and how does this come about? • In what ways do professionals take part in consultations? • In what ways is participation facilitated or blocked through the use of interactional strategies?
Semi-structured interviews	• Studying what people want in terms of participation • Studying what people perceive their roles/participation to be • Identifying what is not voiced in consultations • Identifying global participatory styles or strategies that people say they adopt	• Knowing what actually happened in a specific interaction • Uncovering taken for granted (social/cultural) features of social interaction	• What sort of participation do people want? • What roles do participants say they play, and why? • Are there ways participants would like to have taken part (in a given consultation or in consultations in general) but didn't? Why not?

(*Continued overleaf*)

Table 2.1 *(continued)*

	A more useful method for	*A less useful method for*	*Types of research questions*
Retrospective think aloud	• Studying what people are thinking about at a given point in time • Studying what is not voiced or made explicit in consultations • Understanding aspects of the wider context	• Knowing what actually happened • Understanding how the participants were actually thinking at the time	• What are people thinking about, in relation to their participation in a given sequence? • Are there ways participants might consider taking part but which are blocked? • How do people think about taking part?
Non-participant observation	• Objectively looking at the participation that occurs in consultations and in sequences of interaction • Studying what actually happens in consultations	• Understanding what is going on inside the participants' heads • Knowing what remains unsaid	• What barriers exist to successful patient participation? • In what ways do patients participate and how does this come about?
Focus groups (with moderator)	• Studying what people want in terms of participation • Generating ideas and action points from research • Hearing people's experiences of participation and the effects they report	• Hearing personal experiences (which may not be voiced to a group) • Knowing what actually happened	• What sort of participation do people want? • What are people's experiences in terms of participating in consultations? • How could participation in consultations be facilitated?

outwith the original team commented on the anonymized data. This example draws on one family planning case, in which a patient consulted with a nurse about emergency contraception.

The first data extract, Extract 1, is from an interview in which the nurse talks, in general, about consultation situations in which it may be difficult to share information with patients:

Extract 1 Family planning nurse discussing her perceptions of the difficulties of inviting patients' participation during some consultations

Just say a girl came and she has lower abdominal pain and break-through bleeding, well, I'm think[ing] chlamydia but this is like a new partner or something she's with. Normally I would say, if she was on her own, 'Have you had unprotected sex with several partners?' and they would normally go, 'Yes, you know I've had ten.' But you don't really want to ask that kind of question when the new boyfriend or the husband's sitting in there because that's confidential between us.

(Interview with family planning nurse, A-221)

This extract comes from a semi-structured interview conducted with the nurse prior to recording her consultations. In these interviews, health professionals were asked to talk generally about involving patients in consultations. The extract demonstrates one reported strength of interview data, namely, to access individual's perspectives of a situation or topic which may not be obvious to an external observer (Arksey and Knight 1999). Extract 1 therefore provides some insight into a hypothetical consultation situation, presented by the nurse as an example of the inherent difficulties which confront health professionals when trying to involve, and elicit information from, patients. In this case, the difficulty concerns how the presence of a third party in the room limits patient involvement for reasons of confidentiality. There are also limitations with self-report data, such as this interview example. It does not necessarily demonstrate the actions that may take place in a consultation. That is, this extract does not tell us how a third party's presence may inhibit questions in real clinical scenarios.

The next extract is drawn from a consultation between the nurse in Extract 1 and one of her patients. The nurse and patient have been discussing a range of contraceptive methods that the patient could use (instead of condoms or emergency contraception). In this extract, the nurse raises the possibility of Implanon as an option (lines 1–5). She explains what it is ('a rod', line 5) and the patient registers having heard of it before (line 6). The nurse then describes how successful some people have found it (lines 9–10, 12):

Extract 2 Some evidence of 'difficulty' within the consultation (N = nurse; P = patient)

```
N:  I don't know if you've (.) ever heard of Implanon
    (0.2)
N:  [it's: a::
P:  [Mmm (.) Oh y[es
N:               [A rod
P:  I [have yeah
N:    [Yes (.) and u-
    (0.4)
N:  it's (.) got zero percent failure rate at the moment
    nobody has become pregnant using th[is and a lot of the=
P:                                     [Uh huh
N:  =students are finding it (.) quite useful.
    (1.0)
P:  °Okay°
    (1.2)
N:  Em (.) so it's an option.
```

(Video-recorded nurse–patient consultation in family planning, B-221-453)

This extract was discussed with a conversation analyst researcher who had not been part of the original study team. One feature of particular interest to that researcher was the intervals in talk (lines 13 and 15) that followed the nurse's account of the success of Implanon. Ordinarily, during conversation, turn transition is frequent and quick with few gaps or overlaps (Sacks et al. 1974). In this sequence, the intervals appear long in conversational terms (Jefferson 1985). Previous CA studies have shown how such intervals may display some sort of trouble, reluctance or disagreement that the recipient is having with the preceding talk and in producing a relevant next turn (Davidson 1984; Pomerantz 1984). In relation to health care consultations, several CA studies have offered interpretations of patient silences and their effects on the subsequent interaction (see examples in Stivers 2002; Jones 2003; and Chapter 10 in this volume). There are potentially numerous competing reasons for these intervals. Conversation analysts hesitate to read too much into individuals' internal motives which might 'explain' why these pauses are occurring. Instead, they restrict themselves to noting the presence and effect on the conversation of the silences. In this instance, one effect is the absence of any elaboration or expansion on the part of the patient, beyond her quiet 'Okay', in the intervals during which the nurse also does not talk (lines 13 and 15). Following the second of these intervals, the nurse resumes talk with a tentative summary statement, 'Em so it's an option' (line 16). The discussion subsequently moves to other contraceptive options (injection, pill) and concludes without further mention of the contraceptive rods.

One strength of CA is that it encourages the researcher to consider how participants constantly monitor each other's actions during interaction and how conversational strategies are used, *in situ* by the participants, in 'doing what they are doing, and getting it done' (Schegloff 1992: xviii). In this vein, Extract 2 shows how the patient, through her delayed and minimal response to the nurse's presentation of the Implanon option, contributes to moving the interaction away from further discussion of this type of contraception. Thus, through this sequence, the participants display to each other their understanding of the emerging activities during the consultation: the nurse offers a contraceptive option, the patient refuses to comment or commit, the nurse 'sees' this and moves on to other options.

Further insights were gained when another layer of data and subsequent analysis was added to the interview data in Extract 1 and the consultation data in Extract 2. Specifically, in Extract 3, the patient is responding to a standard think aloud interview prompt, and expresses her thoughts relating to the video clip of Extract 2:

Extract 3 Think aloud interview data illuminating the patient's motives

> She was telling me about . . . rods that they put in the arm and she told me there was so far a 0 per cent failure rate, well, one of my pals is now pregnant with it and I didn't want to tell her that [because] I just felt that it wasn't my place to go around telling, that's my friend's choice . . . And I just feel that it's her decision and how she wants to tackle it because so far they've had a 0 per cent failure chance but now they've not.
>
> (Think aloud interview with woman attending a family planning clinic, D-453)

Through think aloud methods, conscious, but otherwise unspoken, thoughts may be made explicit (Gilhooly and Green 1996; Green and Gilhooly 1996). In this extract, the patient voices her rationale for rejecting rods as an option and for not disclosing her concerns to the nurse. Thus, the researcher gains insight into the patient's motives for not sharing information and into the reasons for the intervals in lines 13 and 15 of Extract 2.

The completeness offered by mixing data of different types, using different research methods and involving an 'external' investigator are immediately obvious at this stage. In Extract 3, the patient offers information that neither of the previous methods had fully captured. When taken individually, the data from each of these methods suggests certain features of patient participation. In combination, they offer the opportunity to build a more coherent picture, by suggesting that there may be occasions in consultations when information is not shared for a variety of reasons. Taking this case as an example, the patient refrained from an opportunity to participate verbally in the consultation (*made apparent through CA*) by withholding her views about rods as a method of contraception. She refrained because she did not want to disclose information that 'belonged' to her friend (*made apparent through think aloud*). This was a situation (withholding information) which, the nurse previously acknowledged (*made apparent through interviews*), may occur in certain contexts during family planning consultations.

We could then argue that, by combining these methods and researchers' perspectives, a deeper understanding was obtained about a feature of patient participation (information sharing) than would have been achieved by any one method or individual researcher alone. Specifically, the analysis strengthens the basis of participation research by providing further detail about patients' contributions to their consultations with nurses (Jarrett and Payne 1995; Caris-Verhallen et al. 1997). It also adds to the debate concerning distinctions between what people say, and what happens in reality (Paley 2001; Miller and Glassner 2004).

Example 2 Cross-study debates

One of our studies (Jones 2005) used a mixed method approach of conversation analysis of audio-recorded interactions and non-participant observation, to study nurse–patient interaction. The data consisted mostly of transcribed examples of nurses managing the interaction in such a way that gave little or no opportunity for patients to express themselves freely or to ask questions (see Chapter 8).

When discussing the data in a seminar, the researcher involved in the study described the findings as an example of 'poor practice' when compared to nursing texts/policies which advocate patient-centred interaction. Others challenged this interpretation, arguing that sometimes patients choose not to share information and are not always dissatisfied with interactions with professionals who managed consultations in such ways (Bugge et al. 2006).

To highlight this point, an interview extract from another of the studies represented in this book is discussed (Extract 4). In this interview, the patient indicated that although he did not know much about his homoeopathic treatment, he did not feel that he wanted to know, or that he needed to question anything further. He reported (prior to the extract shown below) that he was taking because he felt that the GP who prescribed it 'knew what she was doing', and continued:

Extract 4 A patient indicating satisfaction with 'not knowing' about the treatment he is taking

I am still not really that knowledgeable about the whole homoeopathy thing. To be honest, I don't really want to become [knowledgeable] because I think if you learn too much about something you either lose faith in it . . . I was quite happy with the way things went overall, there wasn't anything that I needed to question further.

(Semi-structured interview with patient in homoeopathy, C1-430)

The presentation of findings from different methods gave a conflicting view to the one the researcher had initially adopted of 'poor nursing practice'. This position was challenged by insights into other factors provided by data from other sources. Factors such as a patient's trust in the health professional, and their reluctance to learn too much about a treatment approach, in case they lose faith in it, also influence whether and how the patient has participated (or not) to the level that they desire (and see Chapter 3). These factors need to be considered alongside, and sometimes despite, the actions of the professional.

Example 2 shows how the use of insights from different methods (participant observation and semi-structured interviews), perspectives (patient perspectives from interview accounts and researcher perspectives from participant observation), and contexts can encourage debate about interpretations and findings. Through such debate, researchers are led to question their underlying beliefs and assumptions. This discursive process in turn encourages a broader understanding of participation in health care consultations. Discordant thinking, stimulated by different data, different perspectives and a range of methods, is thus a creative, analytical and interpretive force.

A similar process is reflected in the third and final example, which shows how analytical insights may be confirmed using data drawn from a range of methods.

Example 3 Comparing patient, health professional and researcher perspectives

This example is drawn from a study that used conversation analysis, focus groups and think aloud methods within semi-structured interviews to explore differences between nurses' and doctors' communication with patients in health care consultations (Collins et al. 2003; Collins 2005a). One researcher collected and analysed each of the different types of data, and was therefore in a position to see, hear and compare the various viewpoints (including her own 'researcher perspective').

In Extract 5, a nurse is consulting with a patient about his diabetes. Following the presentation and some discussion of the patient's latest test result which shows a rise in his blood glucose levels, the nurse begins to propose a treatment intervention ('we'll need to do something . . .', line 1):

Extract 5 A nurse being 'open' to a patient's talk (N = nurse; P = patient)

N: but we'll need to do something to bring it down for you
P: yeah
N: uhm (-) and[(you're s-)
P: [shi- I reckon if you took one now,
(1.1)
N: yeah
(0.8)
P: after this last fortnight, (0.5) it would be down
(0.5)
N: right (0.2) right (0.4) and why's that then

(Consultation between a nurse and a patient with diabetes, B-119-338)

Following the patient's minimally expressed agreement ('yeah', line 2), the nurse begins to move on, with 'uhm . . . and . . .'. The nurse stops talking as the patient starts in overlap (lines 3–4). The patient then continues to talk (line 4 onwards) on the prior topic, by elaborating on why his blood glucose levels might have been high at the time of the test. This extract shows that the nurse is responsive to the patient's talk and allows the patient to expand their turn in the conversation.

Extract 6, from a consultation between a doctor and a patient with diabetes, illustrates a different pattern. In conclusion to her description of how she has been feeling since she last visited the doctor, the patient reports a problem of tiredness (line 1):

Extract 6 A doctor moving the talk away from a patient's agenda (D = doctor; P = patient)

P: But otherwise- (.) oth[erwise I'm ↑ti[red.
D: [.hhhhhhh [You're okay. (.)
Okay,

(Consultation between a doctor and a patient with diabetes, B-120-374)

The doctor begins talking during the patient's turn and continues talking beyond the end of it, once the patient has described her problem of tiredness. The doctor's turn, 'you're okay' (line 2), has a closing note to the patient's prior talk: it comes in overlap with the final part of the patient's turn that is projected by 'otherwise'; 'okay' is emphasized and falls to a low pitch at the end. The second 'okay' resumes the business of consulting, projecting further talk. Thus, in contrast to Extract 5, here the doctor's turn moves the talk away from the patient's unresolved 'I'm tired', and back to matters on the doctor's agenda.

Through such comparisons of nurses' and doctors' talk with patients, nurses' communication was found to be characterized by closeness and connectedness with the patient's talk, whereas doctors' communication was characterized by separation and distance from the patients' talk. In focus group discussions that took place once the conversation analyses had been conducted, participants were asked to comment on differences between nurse and doctor communication, prior to hearing the results of the conversation analyses. Extract 7 highlights one nurse's view of the differences:

Extract 7 A nurse commenting on differences between nurses' and doctors' communication

> [Doctors] do seem more experienced in dealing with something and ending the consultation. They don't appear – this might be unfair – to be quite so open to everything. I don't know if nurses are quite so good at finalizing things. We're more open to whatever's wrong with [a patient], and I think because of that, [a patient] might have come in with a sore toe but you get the feeling that 'this woman's depressed', or 'she's more worried about something else', and then you steer the conversation around that.
>
> (Nurse in a focus group, FG3)

Extract 7 builds on the findings from Extracts 5 and 6 by suggesting that nurses may perceive their own professional group to be more open to patients' talk, compared to doctors who may take a narrower focus during consultations with patients. Doctors commented similarly (see Collins et al. 2003). Extract 8 shows a patient's view of differences in communication between doctors and nurses:

Extract 8 A patient accounting for the differences in his communication with doctors and nurses

> When I see [Nurse] I feel I am on the same level as him. [Doctor] is still very approachable but he's still the specialist whereas you're the patient. With [Nurse] you feel that you're working with him equally.
>
> (Patient with multiple sclerosis, in focus group, FG1)

These extracts demonstrate one reported strength of focus group data, namely, to explore opinions in particular as they exist within a social network (Kitzinger and Barbour 1999).

The next extract, from the same study, is from a semi-structured interview with a patient, using think aloud methods. It illustrates how, independently of the conversation analysis, patients articulated their appreciation of the sense of direction in doctors' consultations. This patient commented as follows, on reviewing a video clip from his consultation with an ENT surgeon in a hospital outpatients clinic:

Extract 9 A patient's reflections on characteristics of a doctor's communication in consultations

Every time I had a query he's given me an honest answer straight away, he hasn't had to think about it or ponder it. And that gives me a lot more confidence because he'll give me an answer. And I find that very reassuring in itself. He doesn't have to stop and think 'Oh maybe we'll do this or do that.'

(Patient with a throat cancer in research interview, D1-306)

It is evident, even from these few extracts, that significant stylistic differences appear to exist (Extracts 5 and 6) and are perceived to exist (Extracts 7, 8 and 9) between nurses' and doctors' consultations and that these influence the nature and extent of patient participation.

In this study, findings from the different methods were interwoven to create a deeper understanding about a particular aspect of participation, namely, the different forms of participation that are available when consulting with different professional groups, and to uncover some possible explanations for these differences. The extracts presented illustrate how, at particular junctures when consulting, nurses offered more opportunity for patients to elaborate on a topic or concern, while doctors imparted a sense of direction for the consultation that tended to close conversation on topics that patients may have wished to discuss further (*made apparent through CA*). It can also be seen that health professionals and patients perceived these differences and were able to provide insights into reasons for them (*made apparent through focus groups and through think aloud in interview*). Thus, the convergence of the different perspectives gleaned from the different datasets, and from researcher, patient and health professional perspectives, strengthened understanding about the various forms and dimensions that patient participation can take.

Discussion

Each of the studies in this book, and the examples in this chapter, help us to discover something about patient participation in health care consultations. Sometimes it is individual methods, and at other times a combination of methods, that further our understanding. The insights presented here show

how by combining methods and perspectives we can deepen our understanding of patient participation in health care consultations and improve the scientific rigour in our studies. There are also benefits concerning the development of individual research skills.

How we combined methods to study patient participation

The qualitative methods employed in the studies in this book have some epistemological assumptions in common, as well as being distinct from one another in certain respects. Although working with a mix of methods could have proved a difficult undertaking, the process seemed to work. Due attention was noted of Barbour's (1998) assertions that mixing qualitative methods requires attention to differing epistemologies and simple assumptions of commonality should not be taken for granted.

As our purpose was to reveal a greater understanding of patient participation, differences in perspective, and conflicting findings, were welcomed and used as a means of broadening our knowledge of the concept (Sim and Sharp 1998). We employed various combinations of different methods, investigators, and data on a variety of levels: within study, across study and across disciplines (Denzin 1970). A synergism was achieved through the combination of these approaches, resulting in findings about patient participation and the associated practices of health professionals which seemed to exceed the sum of the individual methods.

Contributions made by this chapter to debates on mixing methods

The advantages and disadvantages of mixing methods within studies are already widely debated (see Shih 1998; Barbour 1999; Razum and Gerhardus 1999). This chapter, we believe, adds two strands to these debates: (1) an analysis of the process through which the benefits are achieved (see pp. 36–7 below, 'The discursive process'), and (2) some evidence of how methods may be productively combined. In particular, we suggest that CA and think aloud techniques, although not natural bedmates in their traditional usage, may be a useful combination under certain circumstances in the study of patient participation. Because CA helps to describe what happens in and through interaction, and 'think aloud' what the participants think happened, and why (and see Pomerantz et al. 1997; Collins 2005b), their combination may result in a more fruitful dialogue between analysts than would otherwise be possible.

Like Foss and Ellefsen (2002), we suggest that findings from different methods are seen as different parts of a knowledge continuum, as opposed to one method being given priority over another. We found that adopting this premise facilitated our own discussions. Furthermore, we believe that such dialogue, that seeks to clarify and refine different viewpoints, results in research findings that health professionals and patients can relate to.

Combining findings across studies

Little has been written about combining findings *across* studies, using mixed methods. Clearly there is evidence of the benefit of combining studies through systematic and general reviews of the literature. What is less well documented is the notion of combining findings by working with the original data and by bringing together different methodological (and hence epistemological) standpoints to give a more complete picture. Even from the limited examples in this chapter we believe we have demonstrated that a greater understanding can be generated than would be the case using any one method. We hope that, as readers progress through the remainder of the book, the insights accrued from the array of methods used will further strengthen this argument.

Cross-disciplinary analyses

Another level of mixing methods and perspectives is across disciplines. The contributors to this book represent a range of professional backgrounds, academic disciplines, and methodological viewpoints. As a result, our data and the concept of patient participation were viewed through different windows, such that the analysts questioned what they saw in different ways. Consequently, in the pursuit of a greater understanding of patient participation, we were made to justify and explain our underlying assumptions, some of which may have otherwise remained deeply embedded, taken for granted, or not fully thought through (and see the Educational Supplement on p. 199).

The discursive process

Each of the above levels of combining methods and perspectives occurred through a discursive research process. This process is crucially different from, for example, reviewing the literature or critically appraising a paper because it offers opportunities to engage with the raw data (the Educational Supplement on pp. 199–202 provides further examples to try yourself). It was as a consequence of this discursive process that the benefits of mixing methods and perspectives for the study of patient participation became manifest. In order for these benefits to surface, it was necessary to make explicit the inherent interpretivist assumption of qualitative methodology, namely, that there is no one objective truth but only a range of constructed truths (Parahoo 1997). Furthermore, we needed to make it explicit that our different methodologies would yield different forms of that constructed truth across a knowledge continuum (Foss and Ellefsen 2002). If the individual contributors to this book had been determined, in discussions, that their findings and methodologies were the only ways of seeing the problem, then it would have been difficult to progress our debates about patient participation. One explanation why the individual contributors may have been able to accept the different forms of emergent truth was because we all worked with qualitative research methods, which depend on critical debate about findings (Barbour 1998). It should be noted that these debates also exist in quantitative circles, and it is therefore possible that mixing quantitative methods would produce similar benefits.

Convergence, discord and uniqueness

We are convinced that by working collaboratively, and sharing data and ideas, a greater understanding of patient participation has been created. This in itself may not be surprising, but what is of interest to us is how this occurred. We would argue that this greater understanding was generated through convergence, discord and uniqueness, and through the juxtaposition and complementarity of different methods.

Convergence could be described as the point where different methods, studies, researchers and/or perspectives identified complementary findings about one dimension of the concept of patient participation. Through their convergence, our understanding of particular dimensions was extended (such as 'information exchange', Example 1; 'different forms of participation with different health professionals', Example 3; and see also extracts in Chapters 5 and 8). This convergence could be considered as a point of overlap between two circles, each representing one method and its findings. The point of overlap between the circles could be viewed (in a three-dimensional way) as cutting down into the circle to demonstrate depth of understanding.

Dissonance between researcher perspectives and methods occurred when different studies generated different findings or explanations for findings. Example 2 is one illustration. In that example, we debated and discussed explanations for the discordance (such as contextual factors). Not only do such explanations represent additional findings about the concept; they also help to highlight differences between the methods employed to study it.

The individual methods also offer their own unique insights. For example, think aloud reflections (Extracts 1 and 9) give voice to patients' viewpoints, while through focus group discussions (Extracts 7 and 8), health professionals' and patients' perceptions about the reasons for differences in communication are made available (and see also Chapter 9 in this volume).

The overlapping of different strands of data and findings creates a more complete three-dimensional picture of patient participation, with the effect of both increasing the surface area of what we know about participation in health care consultations, and the depth to which we understand individual parts of the concept. Overall, this suggests that combining data in the ways described can take us to conceptual and cognitive places that we would not reach with one method, person or dataset.

Improving scientific rigour

Through the process of work being challenged, and encouraging researchers to explain aspects of thinking that may otherwise be taken for granted, we believe that transparency, and hence scientific rigour, are enhanced. In our examples (Example 2, in particular), researchers were encouraged to debate and defend findings with colleagues who, in turn, defended and debated alternate positions. Researchers were thus encouraged to consider participation in a wider context than they may otherwise have done. In addition, through presenting findings, one's inherent (and often subconscious) assumptions could be questioned. These processes can lead to improved transparency, which Guba and Lincoln (1994) have said equates to dependability of the research. The thinking that each of us was encouraged to do, and which was scrutinized by our peers, enabled assumptions to be brought to the fore, for scrutiny by others. These assumptions related both to the concept of participation and to the methods themselves.

Improving researcher skill

Aside from the benefits to research discussed so far, combining methods and perspectives also improved the research ability of individual researchers. In each of the examples presented above, the researchers involved were encouraged to think more widely, both about their own data and about other data in other forms and from other sources. This fosters reflexivity and transparency in conducting research (basic tenets of good research practice, Mays and Pope 2000) and encourages openness to learning about different methods from those with which we each choose to work (and see the Educational Supplement, pp. 199–202).

Applications for communications skills teaching and clinical practice

If, as we have argued, combining methods helps us to understand more and different features about patient participation, clinicians and teachers can similarly use an array of findings from studies that have employed a range of methods to inform their practice or teaching. Although the combination of methods discussed in this chapter may run the risk of antagonizing those who follow a purer research path, there are clear benefits to be gained from combining methods for health care teaching and practice, because of the breadth of discussion and the accessibility of a range of interpretations that such an approach engenders.

Furthermore, the breadth and detail offered here can be helpful in disseminating research to health care professionals, and in reviewing barriers to using research in practice. The utilization of research in practice can be problematic, as it often lacks relevance to 'real' day-to-day work, thus creating a research–practice gap in many areas of health care such as nursing, physiotherapy and psychiatry (Le May et al. 1998; Foster et al. 1999; Parahoo 2000; Young et al. 2001).

The same model for working that has been demonstrated in this chapter in relation to research on patient participation can also be applied to professional education and practice in the field. If clinicians and teachers focus on preferred methods, or those predominantly used in their own profession, they run the risk of not utilizing the full range of understanding that is available in the literature about patient participation in health care consultations.

Conclusion

We have argued that using the methods employed in this book (alone and in combination) can improve the understanding of patient participation in health care consultations, can strengthen scientific rigour in our participation studies and can improve researcher skill. We have suggested that this occurs through a discursive process stemming from concordant, discordant and unique findings yielded from studies that have adopted different methodological standpoints to study the same complex concept. These findings suggest that more opportunity, encouragement and funding for collaborative work at primary and secondary levels of analysis would be beneficial to our understanding of complex concepts and to our academic and professional development. While it may be discomfiting, there are rewards to be gained from seeking out collaborators whose views and assumptions about participation and research are different from our own but who are open to having others interpret their data and confront their assumptions in a constructive way.

Acknowledgement

Some of the material and ideas in this chapter have previously been published as: Jones, A. and Bugge, C. (2006) Improving rigour and understanding through triangulation: an exemplar based on patient participation in interaction, *Journal of Advanced Nursing*, 55(5): 612–21. In that article, further implications for nursing practice and research are detailed.

Recommendations: summary

- In choosing a method of studying patient participation, there are benefits in remaining open to various different possibilities and interpretations, instead of picking the most familiar one.
- In designing research, there is value in exploring the possibilities of investigating a target phenomenon using a combination of methods.
- In studying a complex concept such as patient participation, collaboration with researchers who bring different points of view and who use different methods helps to gain a more concise view of the phenomenon.

PART II
Patient Participation in Practice

3 The meaning of patient involvement and participation in health care consultations

A taxonomy

Andrew Thompson

Commentary

This chapter and Chapter 4 focus on citizens' and patients' views and experiences of patient involvement and participation.

In this chapter, the meaning of patient involvement and participation is explored through reference to empirical evidence from a large-scale qualitative study. The data comprised interviews, focus groups and workshops with participants from different regions across the UK.

For those who took part in this study, participation was viewed as occurring only at a certain level: through the reciprocal relationships of dialogue and shared decision-making between patients and professionals. At another level, many patients support greater involvement in their health care, but not everyone wants to be involved. Patients want professionals to recognize that involvement is optional, and varies according to the particular situation or context (the type of illness, patients' personal characteristics and their relationships with professionals).

From these qualitative data, five different levels of patient-desired involvement are identified: (1) autonomous decision-making; (2) shared decision-making; (3) information-giving/dialogue; (4) information-seeking/receptive; and (5) non-involvement. These are contrasted with professional-determined levels of involvement identified from the literature. By juxtaposing these patient-desired and professional-determined levels of involvement, the dynamic relationship that exists between them comes into view, and the ways in which patients can move from one level of involvement to another are explored.

Identification of these levels, it is argued, provides the basic building blocks for understanding involvement and participation across different contexts, a theme returned to in Chapter 10.

Introduction

The inclusion of patients in health care decision-making, while not new, is currently a policy imperative in many countries and health systems around the world. The belief in patient participation as a desirable goal of health policy has long-standing antecedents at a broad level (WHO 1978). Strongly worded directives or normative statements favouring participation are to be found in a plethora of supranational (WHO 2005), national and sub-national government policy documents. In the UK, neo-liberal administrations since 1979 have made citizen dependency on the State and the paternalism of health care practitioners a target for reforms to encourage a more active consumerist ethos within welfare services (Winkler 1987). Patient choice in service delivery was central to the White Paper *Working for Patients* (Department of Health 1989) and further reinforced in *The Patient's Charter* (Department of Health 1992), which included patients' right to make informed choices. In 1996, the Government launched the *Patient Partnership Strategy* (NHS Executive 1996), which explicitly recognized the need for patient involvement in decisions about their own care.

Since 1997, the New Labour Government could be viewed as being in the vanguard of promoting citizen involvement through its modernization agenda of inclusiveness, stakeholder engagement and partnership working (Department of Health 1997; 1998). The expected benefits of involvement were laid out in *Patient and Public Involvement in the New NHS* (Department of Health 1999), including improvements in service quality, care outcomes and population health. In England, the strategic *NHS Plan* (Department of Health 2000) emphasized the need for a health service responsive to the needs of patients, lay carers and the public, expecting those on the receiving end of care to take an active part. Better opportunities for patient and lay carer involvement in health care delivery and access to relevant information were key recommendations of the critical Bristol Royal Infirmary Inquiry Report (UK Parliament 2001a). Subsequently, the Health and Social Care Act (UK Parliament 2001b) made it a legal requirement to involve patients and the public. Recently, patient choice of hospital and treatment has been made central to the marketization of health services in England (Department of Health 2003).

Two distinct approaches to the involvement of patients can be discerned that reflect contrasting political values, one espousing individual freedom to make choices and the other a more collective freedom to achieve inclusiveness and equity. The former, consumerist model places health service users in the role of mimicking customers in market-style relationships (Mullen and Spurgeon 2000), exemplified in the current emphasis on patient choice of hospital in England. Williams and Grant (1998) believe that this contradicts the meaning of person-centredness, while Thompson (1995) argues that it negates their role as co-producers of their own health and health care, not to mention their democratic role as co-owners in the British NHS. The latter approach emphasizes the democratic dimension of quality (Pfeffer and Coote 1991), requiring a developmental process of engagement over time, such as involving the voluntary sector in hospital boards. However, individual actions are not necessarily consumerist, nor collective actions necessarily democratic (Lupton et al. 1998). Both approaches lay stress on patient empowerment, in the former case resting on the power of 'exit' when dissatisfied, or the making of complaints with compensatory redress when there is no alternative, and in the latter case relying on 'voice' to exert change more directly (Hirschman 1970). Emanuel and Emanuel (1997) see these models as exemplifying the conflict between an economic and a political model of health care, although in essence they are both politically driven.

We can identify other influences on the patient–professional relationship within health care encounters. One is a notable increase in lay knowledge about health care and forms of self-help. Olszewski and Jones (1998) identify the steady growth of information outside formal health services, through voluntary group books/leaflets, help-lines, and, more recently, use of the Internet (Eysenbach 2000). In tandem with recent scandals and negative media reporting, this may be fuelling an increased awareness of health professionals' fallibility and uncertainties in diagnoses, linked to increasing scepticism towards medicine and science (Beck 1992). In part, this also reflects increasing acknowledgement of wider influences on health (Acheson 1998), as well as increasing evidence of disparities in clinical practice for similar conditions (Wennberg 2002). A further important contributory factor has been the shift within post-industrialized countries from a focus on acute conditions to chronic health problems requiring continuous and complex management (McEwan et al. 1983; Holman and Lorig 2000). This has led to policy recognition in the *Expert Patients Programme* (Department of Health 2001) of the important contribution made by people with chronic conditions to the management of their own health care. It is this perceived 'partnership of equals between patients and professionals' that encourages Hunter (2004: 52) to see potential change in the power imbalance between 'repressed' citizens and the 'dominant' professionals or 'challenging' managers (Alford 1975). There is also pressure to increase accountability (Barnes 1997) and to democratize publicly-run health systems (Hogg 1999), although some cynically view participation as a device to co-opt patients into unpalatable rationing decisions (White 2000). Finally, there is a discernible shift towards incorporating patients' perceptions, values and preferences into a more subjective medicine, moving health care goals towards quality of life and patients' perceptions of health (Sullivan 2003).

Models of involvement and participation in consultations

The terminology describing patients taking an active part in their consultations with professionals includes 'involvement' and 'participation'. These concepts are often used synonymously, without a clear understanding of their difference, despite being problematized individually (Elwyn et al. 2000; Jones et al. 2004). In a notable exception, Cahill (1996) distinguished patient participation from the precursor concepts of involvement (basic, often delegated tasks) and collaboration (intellectual co-operation) and the ultimate concept of partnership (joint venture). Patient participation requires a narrowing of the information/competence gap between professional and patient, with some surrendering of power by the professional which conveys benefit to the patient, even if there is no consensus.

Early conceptualization of the patient–doctor relationship outlined a hierarchy of patient control from passivity to participation (Szasz and Hollender 1956), since when ideas of shared decision-making and patient autonomy have come to the fore (Coulter 2002). Charles and DeMaio (1993) proposed a framework, based on Arnstein (1969), in which patient involvement is identified as occurring at one of three levels of increasing patient power: consultation, partnership, or lay control. These levels are reflected in four of the currently most discussed models of treatment decision-making: *paternalism*, where the professional knows best and patient involvement is limited to being given information or giving consent; *shared decision-making*, where both the process and the outcome of decisions about treatment options are shared between patient and professional; *professional-as-agent*, where professionals possess the technical expertise, but patient preferences are incorporated into their decision-making; and, *informed decision-making*, where the technical expertise is transferred to the patient, who makes the final decision (Charles et al. 1997; Coulter 1997). Combining these four levels with the exclusionary levels of manipulation/therapy identified by Arnstein (1969), we can conceive of professional-determined patient involvement along the power continuum shown in Figure 3.1.

While there is some agreement about different models of patient involvement and the different conditions that would appear to favour each, much research has been limited to certain types of patient in consultation with doctors, often focused on treatment decisions, rather than broader considerations of citizens (as past, current and potential patients), health care professions, or purposes of consultations. Moreover, the impression gained is of a normative perspective driven by professionals. However (and see Rogers 1989), it is important to reflect current meanings as embodied in patients' own understandings of these concepts within specific contexts. As Guadagnoli and Ward

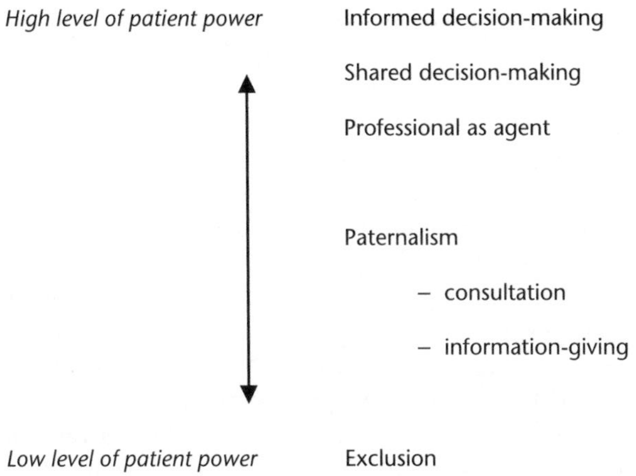

Figure 3.1 Professional-determined patient involvement.

(1998: 337) conclude, 'Participation should be defined by whatever level the patient is most comfortable with.'

In recognition of these trends, pressures and policy shifts, this chapter aims to explore the extent and contexts in which patients themselves are desirous of greater opportunities for voice, rather than exit, within health care consultations, centred on an empirical study of patient and citizen views of their preferences. From a synthesis of this material with existing literature on professional views of patient involvement, a taxonomy of involvement and participation within consultations will be constructed to offer conceptual clarity and as a means of enabling health care practitioners and managers to understand the dynamics and realities of patient-centred policy.

Methods

This is an exploratory, qualitative study based on a deliberative design, with a subset of individuals asked to discuss their views more than once. In Phase I of the study, 48 semi-structured interviews were planned, with participants recruited from three GP surgeries in northern England, reflecting age (18–25, 35–55, 70+), gender and presence/absence of chronic disease.

In Phase II, 36 focus groups were planned with three different types of citizens in three areas in northern England and three areas in southern England. One type comprised 24 homogeneous groupings of individuals, unaffiliated to any voluntary/community groups, reflecting combinations of age, gender and disease, as in Phase I. Those interviewed in Phase I were included here in six of their own groups. The two other types were drawn from local voluntary organizations/community groups: six had a specific interest in health and six did not.

In Phase III, 12 workshops were planned with the same groups as in Phase II: all unaffiliated citizens together (age and gender) and, separately, all voluntary/community group members together in each of the six areas.

Table 3.1 shows the actual response rates, generating 208 individuals in total. While nearly all the groups met, the recruitment of individuals was difficult and declined over the phases.

The geographical areas and GP surgeries were chosen to reflect social class differences within different types of physical environment (as a proxy for access): two rural areas that contrasted relative wealth (south-east) and poverty (north-east); two suburban areas with mixed levels of wealth and deprivation; and two inner cities characterized by high levels of deprivation. Access was negotiated with each GP surgery (five multi-practitioner and one single-handed) and ethical approval was given by relevant ethics committees.

Sampling was theoretically driven to derive a broad range of opinions, with age, gender, ethnicity, social class, health needs and experience chosen as the most discriminating variables. For pragmatic reasons, participation in this research was limited to adults who could communicate in English, irrespective of ethnicity. Having a chronic condition was believed to offer the best proxy for the presence of health needs and NHS experience. Individuals opted in by confirming agreement to an invitation letter from their GP.

One member from eight local voluntary/community groups in each area was invited to attend. Groups representing minority ethnic populations were given priority in selection, where possible. Those who were members of several voluntary groups were asked to speak on behalf of the group from which they had been invited. Paid workers employed in any voluntary group were specifically excluded.

All focus group discussions and workshops were held either in the local GP surgery or a location neutral to the participants, with times arranged to suit the majority, and participants receiving remuneration for each meeting they attended, to cover travel expenses and care for dependants. All interviews and focus group discussions were tape-recorded and verbatim transcriptions were made for entering into qualitative software (Nud*ist 4) prior to analysis.

Within a broader set of issues for discussion, all respondents were asked to consider their desired type of involvement and that of the public in general at the service delivery level of decision-making. Additional personal and group information was recorded (via self-completion questionnaires for the focus groups).

The combination of individual interviews and focus groups allowed a more deliberative understanding to develop among the respondents, as well as offering the benefits of group dynamics and more personal reflections to form a blend of public and private accounts to inform the analysis (Silverman 1993;

Table 3.1 Response rates to each phase of the research

		Phase I	*Phase II*		*Phase III*	
		Interviewed individuals	*Individuals*	*Focus groups*	*Individuals*	*Workshop groups*
Unaffiliated Individuals	Northern areas only	44 →	29	6	63	6
	All areas		82	16		
Voluntary/Community Groups	Health		43	6	58	6
	Non-health		36	6		
Total		44	190	34	121	12
Response rate (%)	Individuals	92	58		37	
	Groups			94		100

Note: n = 208.

Morgan 1997; Chapter 2 in this volume). Individuals were chosen from voluntary/community groups, some with greater experience of the NHS, to learn of their collective organizational perspectives on involvement. Unaffiliated individuals were put together to encourage those less experienced to feel safe to explore ideas and opinions through working in groups of similar personal characteristics, thus avoiding, for example, conflicts between genders or age groups.

The transcripts were thematically coded and analysed by incorporating a combination of categories derived initially from the topic guides for the interviews and focus groups and supplemented or refined with those that emerged spontaneously within these meetings. Due to the voluminous quantity of data, a small sub-sample of text was coded and checked by two researchers. Cross-cutting comparative analyses were conducted by several members of the research team, which helped to triangulate the findings. The evidence presented below is drawn from individuals' views, as past, current or potential patients, of involvement in consultations only, from Phases I and II, with respondent face validity confirmed through gauging responses to feedback of initial results in Phase III. Evolving understanding of the concepts and their contextual conditions were discussed and refined within the research team and after various seminar presentations. Quotations have been selected according to three criteria: (1) illustrative of a particular theme; (2) offering a range of views where there was heterogeneity; and (3) being focused and succinct.

Results

Overall views of involvement

Unaffiliated individuals' views emanated from direct experiences of self/dependants; second-hand experiences of family, friends, or community contacts; and the media. Involvement for them included one or more of: information, explanations, openness, communication, shared knowledge, emotional care, exploration of choices, dialogue and decision-making. In addition to the above sources, voluntary sector representatives drew from members of their group or cause. Health voluntary groups especially had clear views of the meaning of involvement, including, in addition to the above list, building partnerships and access for all.

Participation in consultations was broadly understood as involving patients in discussions about their condition, providing them with relevant information, asking for their opinion on possible treatments, and involving them in the decision-making process, should they so wish. Many noted that not everyone aspires to being involved at all times and in all situations. This emphasis on rights rather than obligations parallels participation literature in other contexts (UNICEF 2001).

The findings are presented to illustrate the range of degrees of involvement which participants desired, depending on their own context.

Expressions of desire for involvement

Various reasons were advanced as to why some people could not be involved, including emergency conditions, psychological distress and level of cognitive ability, for which relative youth, dementia and head injuries were examples. Many respondents specifically mentioned lay carers, who were deemed to offer substitute or complementary involvement on occasions. The wide sample range of types of citizen presents a rich diversity of views on involvement. However, there appeared to be a high degree of unanimity about the existence of different levels of involvement and participation, whatever the personal proclivities. These levels are now presented in relation to patients' relative power to influence decisions.

Non-involvement

Some, often with limited experience of health care, expressed trust in professionals to do the best for them, showing faith in their knowledge and abilities derived from years of education and training:

> **Extract 1**
> [In] the past I've always, even with the kids, tended to leave it up to the doctor because at the end of the day he's the one who makes the decision and you've got to trust his decision, but I've never had a case where a doctor's suggested something and I've had to turn round and say 'Not a cat in hell's chance.'
> (Middle-aged man, little experience, northern suburbs, interview)

However, as the following extract reveals, greater experience of a negative kind leads to a contrary position:

> **Extract 2**
> Respondent 1: I think it depends a lot on how much trust you've got in the medical establishment and, like, from my personal [and] family's experience . . . there's been a lot of mistakes and things made by doctors that have resulted in, like, my dad, for one, dying . . . So . . . it forces you to have an opinion of the medical profession, I suppose.
> Respondent 2: Do you think that's made you want to get more involved with any treatment, that experience?

Respondent 1: Yeah, definitely. And, well, not just that but not to trust doctors so much as if . . . they're always right . . . but to just be a bit more wary about anything.

(Younger men, northern inner city, focus group)

For others it was more a case of wanting to trust, as a way of coping with fear and reducing anxiety:

Extract 3

I would just like to trust me doctor . . . I don't want to know what's wrong with us, you know. No, I don't, I really don't, cos I'm terrified . . . so I would sooner just think to meself, 'Well, me doctor's . . . trustworthy . . . to put us right.'

(Middle-aged woman, rural north-east, focus group)

Part of the explanation for trusting professionals appears to reflect a lack of medical knowledge in patients, suggesting low self-confidence or relatively low valuation of their own knowledge:

Extract 4

[P]eople don't know . . .; they're not educated in the things that can go wrong with you . . . we put our faith in the doctors and we accept everything that they tell us and I think . . . we can only be involved to an extent, because if the doctor tells us something and it's . . . very high-faluted, or something that's very technical that we don't understand, then . . . there's not really a lot of point in telling us as far as decision-making.

(Younger woman, rural south-east, focus group)

There were many indications that the responsibility of involvement could be burdensome, which probably explains why having the choice to be involved or not has been strongly emphasized:

Extract 5

He was diagnosed ten days before he died, right. Well, he didn't know he had it and, to me, for someone who thinks they know best to go and tell him that he had it, did he want, was he responsible? Was he in a fit state for it to be thrust on him? . . . To take responsibility for this, it's enormous.

(Health voluntary groups, northern inner city, focus group)

Some clearly saw this responsibility as either life-shortening or requiring unwarranted effort:

Extract 6

I know that when my husband was very ill we never talked about the illness, never and he lived about four years longer than he should have done quite happily.

(Older woman, rural south-east, focus group)

Extract 7

Respondent:	. . . like I say, if it works and stuff, cool; if it doesn't, go back to the doctor and say that's not working.
Moderator:	But you don't really want to know any more than that?
Respondent:	Not really.
Moderator:	Why not, do you think?
Respondent:	. . . laziness.

(Younger man, northern inner city, focus group)

Others were referred to, often including younger people, who felt alienated from the NHS (and other official bodies) and had difficulties relating to the concept of involvement:

Extract 8

[A]lcoholics or people like that . . . the fact that they may have some say in their own treatment is completely alien to them . . . cos they've been pushed around and downtrodden by every single official body that they come across . . . The fact that they could have a say, will have some kind of input to their own health issues, hasn't really dawned on a lot of them; they haven't even thought of it as a concept.

(Non-health voluntary groups, inner London, focus group)

Information-seeking / Information-receptive

The following person expressed the view that being given information is a normative expectation and that being receptive to such information is an elementary stage of involvement:

Extract 9

[Y]ou're involved by actually being told what they think the diagnosis is, what the options, the side effects is. In the end there may be no option, as it were but at least the fact you've been told . . . as opposed to . . . twenty years ago you were lucky if you came out clutching a prescription not knowing what the hell it was going to do.

(Middle-aged man, northern suburbs, focus group)

However, for many, this did not contain the vital ingredient of involvement:

Extract 10
They could always just give you a leaflet and say, 'You know that's what's wrong with you, that's what we're giving you, blah-de-blah, and you can go', but you know there's no contact there. I wouldn't say they're involving a patient. They're just informing them. It's not really what you want here.

(Younger man, northern inner city, focus group)

Understanding the presenting illness or condition was a core requirement:

Extract 11
I'd want to know all the information, but I don't know about me necessarily playing much of an active role in it, cos I'm a bit sort of trusting really. So, if a doctor gives me medicine, I'll take it.

(Middle-aged woman, northern inner city, focus group)

Furthermore, many felt that information provided a means to maintain some control over their lives:

Extract 12
I think that the key to anything, in terms of being ill or needing treatment, is your own ability to control that situation and so, therefore, I think you have to have a part to play in that . . . I think that's crucial to the doctor–patient relationship that you play a role and I know I personally would be unhappy with just being told what to do. That's not to say that I don't defer to the professionalism and the skills, but generally I'm happier if somebody explains things to me or I feel the environment is conducive to actually asking things I don't understand and asking the possible consequences of something that's wrong with me.

(Middle-aged woman, northern inner city, focus group)

It was also clear that information was a basic building block for decision-making:

Extract 13
It's very difficult because one has to be, to a certain degree, knowledgeable about the variety of treatments that are available and well versed in the complications of the condition that you may be suffering from. Then you can make a judgement . . . I think that there should be more information . . . freely available . . . in health centres which deal with the understanding of illness rather than treatment of illness.

(Middle-aged woman, inner London, *de facto* interview[1])

Information-giving / Dialogue

Greater confidence in self-knowledge and the need to be listened to and heard exemplify this level:

> **Extract 14**
> I think that they should treat you as if you do know what you're talking about. You're the one that's feeling ill and they should actually . . . 'Well, how are you feeling and do you think that it could be something, or something else?'
> (Middle-aged woman, London suburbs, focus group)

The chance to explore choices was recognized as requiring discussion, even if it did not lead on to making decisions:

> **Extract 15**
> To have, I suppose, informed choice. To be able to have that choice whether to make the decision and to discuss it with somebody who knows all the information and knows the consequences and the risks and to say 'Well, if it comes down to it, I trust you.' And I suppose they'd have overall say, because they know more about it than I do, but I would like to be involved with that and be given as much information myself to at least say 'No, I don't want that', rather than just saying 'Yeah, I'll do whatever.'
> (Younger woman, little experience, northern suburbs, interview)

Linked to this discussion was a need for greater openness and honesty from professionals:

> **Extract 16**
> . . . more open and much more honest. But in the end I don't want them to hide behind their professional competence, that I am just as competent at what I do as they are with what they do, so in furtherance of this discussion more honesty, more information and, if it is of a highly technical nature, surely they are intelligent enough to explain it to me. And if it's beyond my understanding, please write it down and I will get it translated.
> (Non-health voluntary groups, northern inner city, focus group)

Where professionals were prepared to be open to two-way communication, there was recognized to be a greater chance of rapport and reciprocity in the relationship:

Extract 17

You've got to feel like you're going in and having a discussion rather than them telling you and asking questions and you're just sat there answering. Yeah, you've got to get some form of rapport, haven't you?

(Younger woman, northern suburbs, focus group)

Shared decision-making

Here respondents wished to exercise an informed choice, being guided and allowed to express opinions in partnership with professionals:

Extract 18

I think we're talking about informed choice, so if people are going to be involved in their own health care, then it does mean that somebody else has got to take the time to explain to them what is actually wrong with them and what . . . choices there are for putting it right and then some people get involved in it and feel a part of a team deciding their own future. So I think it's a team, which might be just you and the GP, or it might be you and a wider group of people . . . but the key to me is the person feeling that they themselves and their opinions are valued in decision-making.

(Health voluntary groups, inner London, focus group)

This sharing of decisions was believed to lead to better decisions being made:

Extract 19

[T]he last two serious occasions I've gone into the doctor's I've actually told him what I think is wrong. One occasion he's disagreed with me and then been proved that I was right, which is bad news, and on the second occasion he was fabulous, you know, and it was great, 'We've got to do this X, Y and Z' and it's because you're sharing the same information.

(Middle-aged man, rural south-east, focus group)

While it can be viewed very positively, reasons for desiring involvement at this level can also be an expression of mistrust:

Extract 20

Moderator: Do you think that patients should be involved in decisions about their own care and treatment?

Respondent: Yes . . . because, very often, I believe that the medical profession and hospitals in particular are very structured societies and they're more interested with the kind of world that they've built up and the control that they can exert than the care of their patients.

(Middle-aged woman, inner London, *de facto* interview[2])

Autonomous decision-making

While there appeared to be relatively little support for independent decision-making, probably related to concerns about the high degree of concomitant responsibility, there were some who believed they had equal or even superior knowledge about their condition, typically those living with chronic illness:

Extract 21

With my diabetes they tell me one thing and I'll do something else. Because if you're living with diabetes you know yourself when your sugar's gone and you know when your sugar's too high . . . I don't tell her [diabetic nurse] nothing . . . She doesn't listen . . . I told her the other day I had two hypos in one day and she told me to higher up me insulin. You know you just don't do that. So I stayed to what I was taking anyway . . . cos I know when I feel good.

(Middle-aged woman, northern inner city, focus group)

Some preferred to be able to manage their condition themselves:

Extract 22

You know I made a decision to have surgery and radiation but not chemotherapy . . . I'd read around it a lot and found various advice agencies and I was quite informed . . . There's a lot of people who's having a really hard time with chemo and stuff like that . . . because they see the doctors as the experts . . . rather than managing their own disease.

(Middle-aged man, northern inner city, focus group)

Extract 23

I think I want . . . an advised choice . . . I just generally go and have a chat and we sort of say, 'Well, do you think we should do this?' and . . . I don't leave it to the doctor. I have an input definitely and in the end I make the final decision. I have been known to sort of play around with my doses with my asthma things as well without consulting a doctor, just because I think I know and it seemed to work.

(Younger woman, much experience, northern suburbs, interview)

Some respondents had an even broader view of health care that extended beyond the traditional reaches of professionals:

Extract 24

Health care isn't . . . purely about managing health problems because it has a knock-on effect into social aspects of people's lives . . . [P]eople should have a large amount of say in how they conduct their lives in view of the disabilities, or despite the disabilities in a lot of cases.

(Non-health voluntary groups, rural north-east, focus group)

Developing a taxonomy

Through linking positive and negative opinions about how citizens would like to be involved, it has been possible to develop a taxonomy with five discrete levels of *patient-desired involvement* in consultations, as shown in Table 3.2. Those levels that can be achieved through self-determination are hereafter labelled as *patient-determined involvement.* While this suggests an active role, the amount of involvement that patients wish to have might be more subtle and reflect an internalized set of normative expectations about their right to receive information, whether demanded or not. Patient involvement in this scenario might depend on how much effort they perceive it to require and how much they are prepared to exert to satisfy those expectations. In other words, apparently passive positions adopted by patients can belie a potential for more assertive articulation of involvement, should it be deemed appropriate and worthwhile. The taxonomy also recognizes that some may not wish to be involved due to vulnerability, lack of interest, or apathy, although even for these patients it may represent a deliberate act of detachment, or even defiance, in the face of perceived social or personal exclusion.

Table 3.2 Levels of involvement

Patient-desired level	*Patient-determined*	*Co-determined (Participation)*	*Professional-determined*
4	Autonomous decision-making		Informed decision-making
3		Shared decision-making	Professional-as-agent
2	Information-giving	Dialogue	Consultation
1	Information-seeking/receptive		Information-giving
0	Non-involved		Exclusion

By comparing this taxonomy with existing theories of patient involvement, five parallel, although meaningfully different, levels of *professional-determined involvement* can be aligned with it, representing how professionals attempt to position patients within consultations. These begin from two paternalistic positions of excluding patients (level 0) or simply giving them information considered necessary by professionals (level 1). Consultation (level 2) is used in the Arnstein (1969) sense of lacking any requirement to reflect the patient's agenda or to act on the findings. The professional-as-agent model (level 3) denotes the incorporation of patients' views and preferences with their own expertise to make the final decisions, which necessitates some prior consultation or dialogue, while informed decision-making (level 4) involves professionals giving their expertise to patients to decide for themselves.

Where patients desire to be involved in dialogue or the sharing of decisions, this can only be effected through a matching willingness by professionals, labelled here as *co-determined involvement*, or, reflecting the overall views outlined earlier, *participation*. Dialogue, although occurring at the same level as patients wanting to give information, or professionals asking patients what they think, requires the added component of two-way communication within conditions of openness and mutual respect. Dialogue is seen to underpin the possibility of shared decision-making, although it may be that patients would rather the professional (as agent) took the final decision, based on knowledge of their views and preferences. Participation does not, therefore, necessarily include the sharing of decisions or, by implication, a consensus.

Each level represents a relative position of patient power between the extremes of non-involvement or exclusion (notwithstanding the possible powerful intent of self-exclusion) and full autonomy. This is not to say that more power is necessarily more desirable, since there is a concomitant increase in responsibility for the outcomes, which some would find insupportable. It is assumed that moving up each level beyond non-involvement is typically dependent upon each preceding level having been sufficiently achieved for a particular situation, although this could easily alter when faced with different professionals, settings or illnesses, or between different types of consultation activity (see Chapters 1 and 6 in this volume). It is conceivable that patients might make the jump from level 1 to level 4, should they wish for any reason to make decisions without recourse to professionals. However, since use of NHS services requires professional sanction, this could effectively exclude them from formal health care and would be unlikely without much experience at other levels. Nonetheless, full autonomy, it is believed, can mean that patients act with or without any information derived from professionals. The resultant position in which patients are located will depend on their relative power and the willingness of professionals to adapt to them.

Moving between the levels

Despite respondents having clear views about their desired level of involvement, it was usually qualified by a number of determining characteristics, reflecting three distinct contextual dimensions. First, there are two attributes which reflect the nature of the health care need itself: the type of illness, whether it is acute or chronic, with the latter offering greater possibilities for involvement due to prolonged experience:

> **Extract 25**
> [A] chronic disease like, say, diabetes, as you grow up, your knowledge increases so . . . you know your diabetes probably as well as any doctor . . . that way they don't have to trust somebody else so much . . . because they can take control of it. But . . . acute illness information can be given, but the patient doesn't have a chance to develop . . . the knowledge that the doctor has, so then you know involvement is going to be more limited.
> (Younger man, London suburbs, focus group)

Or due to the seriousness of the condition, which is related to the degree of expert knowledge:

> **Extract 26**
> Well . . . things that aren't life-threatening in my view would be something that you have a say in. If something's life-threatening, you have to hope that you'd be told what to do and it would be the right thing to do . . . It's really, in my view, about if you've got a choice that can be made on a sort of personal, social level, as opposed to on a medical level, then you should be involved in it . . . Involvement reduces [for serious illness] but I would say information needs to increase.
> (Younger man, London suburbs, focus group)

Second, there are the personal characteristics of patients, which in part are likely to reflect socio-demographic variables, linked to knowledge and experience, and personality:

> **Extract 27**
> [I]t has to be . . . a balance between what the individual's personality and character wants and what the overall service should be doing in recognizing individual choice, but being open to that . . . changing, so the person who showed no interest might then say, 'Hang on, now I actually want to engage much more seriously.'
> (Health voluntary groups, inner London, focus group)

Third, there is the patient–professional relationship, characterized by trust, which gives confidence to allow others to act on our behalf:

Extract 28

Throughout my life I've always had competent GPs and they've always been really helpful . . . we get on well and that sort of thing. So it's easier to trust someone and trust their decision . . . But if I was in a new situation where I didn't know my GP, or a new area, that sort of thing, then I would want to know a lot more about what was going on and what was being said.

(Younger man, London suburbs, focus group)

Trust features where there is little patient experience or knowledge, or where seriousness increases the possibility of decision-making regret. Situations which question this trust can be the spur for greater involvement, until trust can be established or restored, at which point it is conceivable that continued demand for involvement would be less strong. However, trust which emerges through greater involvement may create the conditions for a sustained desire for involvement, as self-confidence and competence grow and mature. The demand for involvement appears to reflect a combination of these dimensions, as outlined in Table 3.3.

Table 3.3 Dynamic dimensions of involvement

	Reduced demand	*Increased demand*
Need for health care		
Type of illness	acute	chronic
Seriousness	high	low
Personal characteristics		
Knowledge/experience	(variable)	(variable)
Personality	passive	active
Professional relationship		
Trust	high	low

Discussion

Amid the extensive range of views in this study, we can identify five distinct levels of patient involvement in consultations. These levels provide a set of building blocks between basic demands for more information and the ability to share or control decisions about health care, while acknowledging that some patients in some contexts would prefer not to be involved at all. The main distinguishing feature between patient involvement and patient participation concerns the degree to which patients take part in the decision-making process. The same patient may wish to be involved at different levels in relation to different circumstances and it may change over time for the same person in the same context (see the Educational Supplement, pp. 203–4, for an exercise which relates this to your own experiences). Patient involvement is, therefore, a complex, multi-faceted and dynamic concept for which this taxonomy offers a necessary simplification to assist professionals, managers, or policy-makers to respond appropriately.

While there are clear parallels with the work of Arnstein (1969) and others, those levels reflect a concern and perspective that emanate from professionals, rather than, as here, patients themselves. This study combined individual interviews with focus groups to generate a rich, narrative understanding of how citizens view involvement and participation in health care delivery. Evidence of construct validity is indicated by the study issues reflecting much of what is already known, while the breadth of the sampling has allowed greater insight into the similarities and differences between and within the 'activists' and 'non-activists' in a way that broadens and deepens our understanding of the complexity of the concept. Those who participated may not have been typical of the general public and they may have been more in favour of involvement. Nonetheless, we have been able to discern a wide variety of viewpoints that enable us to establish the likely range of opinions, including those opposed to involvement. A more quantitative approach would be required to determine the distribution of views across the various publics.

For some purposes a more sophisticated delineation of levels of involvement may be required, such as disaggregating the stages involved in the information process, or incorporating the time dimension within and between various episodes of care (Gafaranga and Britten 2003). There is also a need to see how such a taxonomy would work with different kinds of therapeutic relationship, contrasting those of the conventional allopathic variety, largely explored here, with other forms that emphasize patient-constituted relationships, such as psychoanalysis and homoeopathy (see Peräkylä and Vehviläinen 2003; Chapters 5 and 7 in this volume). Despite the broad scope of this study, a consequential limitation has been a lack of attention to in-depth analysis of specific conditions or contexts. The literature partly addresses these, but there is a dearth of evidence from many health care encounters. It is also clear that, despite identifying some socio-demographic differences, significant gaps exist in our understanding of how different ethnic groups perceive involvement. The impact of personality, particularly the emotional disposition to illness, also needs further research.

Hoggett (2001), in warning of the dangers of typologies that characterize individuals, suggests the use of continuums of agency and reflexivity, which explore relative powerlessness and the complexities of choice, to see how roles change over time. We also need to study the social and political contexts that give power, morality and meaning to patient involvement (Glenister 1994). Reflecting these, this taxonomy offers a way of identifying the contexts that enable patients to determine their own desired level of involvement, as an expression of voice within consultations.

In conclusion, many patients support greater involvement in service delivery, but they want professionals to recognize that this needs to be optional and varies according to the context and probably over time too. Maintenance of trust appears to be crucial, with its erosion likely to lead to increased demand for involvement, although it might also lead to self-exclusion. Participation, when it is the ideal form of relationship, requires professionals to engage in two-way communication and effectively share the power they undoubtedly have with their patients on the basis of mutual respect and openness.

The proposed taxonomy identifies the different perspectives on involvement and offers a means to link the two. In this way, this study enables an understanding of how involved patients wish to be within different aspects of a consultation and why, alongside professional preferences, offering the possibility of a mutually acceptable arrangement, facilitating more effective communication from professionals and satisfying patients as a result.

Notes

1. Focus group with one attendee.
2. Ditto.

Acknowledgements

Especial thanks to colleagues in the Health in Partnership project on which this chapter is based, including Kai Rudat, Sophie Staniszewska, Marcia Kelson, David Gilbert, Sara Bruce, Emily Gray, Malcolm McCrae, Susan Levy and Marilyn Kendall, as well as the Department of Health for funding the research. Grateful thanks also to Rosa Suñol, Carol Bugge and Sarah Collins for helpful comments in making the taxonomy clearer.

This chapter has been reprinted from *Social Science & Medicine* (2007), Thompson AGH, The meaning of patient involvement and participation in health care consultations: a taxonomy. *Social Science and Medicine* 64: 1297–1310, Copyright (2006), with permission from Elsevier.

Recommendations: summary

- Patient participation, as understood by many members of the public, is a specific form of involvement that implies a reciprocal relationship of dialogue, and potentially shared decision-making, with health care professionals.
- Involvement in consultations ranges from information-seeking/ information-receptiveness to autonomous decision-making.
- Not all members of the public would want to be involved during a health care consultation for a wide variety of reasons.
- Demand for involvement is dynamic, reflecting in part the type of illness and its seriousness, the knowledge/experience and personality of the patient, and the degree of trust patients have in their relationship with the professional.
- Interviews and focus groups allow a narrative approach to be used to construct meaning in the health care consultation from the varied experiences and expectations of the public, as patients or members of voluntary/community groups.

4 What is a good consultation and what is a bad one?

The patient perspective

Fiona Stevenson

Commentary

Similar to the approach taken in Chapter 3, this chapter explores patients' observations in interviews about their experiences of consultations; particularly, patients' judgements of 'good' or 'bad' in relation to general practice consultations. These data are used to reflect on patients' expectations concerning participation and involvement in their health care.

While there is a generally held assumption that patient participation makes for better consultations, the perspectives of patients as to what makes a consultation 'good' or 'bad', and what these might tell us about participation, have been little explored.

From the views expressed in this study, patients' judgements as to what makes a consultation 'good' or 'bad', and the extent to which it enlists their participation, were seen to vary. Their evaluations seemed to be dependent on notions of participation or involvement. Patients were generally positive about consultations in which opportunities for participation were available, and negative about consultations in which opportunities for participation appeared to be blocked. The doctor's behaviour was regarded as crucial, in creating the conditions for patient participation, and there was only limited discussion of shared responsibilities and of patients' behaviours.

This chapter makes two distinct contributions to understanding what participation means and how it works in practice. First, by drawing on research interviews conducted with patients following their consultations, these data provide insights into what actually happened, with reference to particular consultations. Second, as these data were not collected specifically to study participation, the responses can be viewed as a form of evaluation which reveals people's thoughts on participation without having to ask them directly what it means.

Introduction

In recent decades, there has been a notable shift in the relationship between doctors and patients, as documented in the academic literature. Until the 1970s a strongly doctor-centred model of the clinical encounter held sway, in which the epistemological authority of medical knowledge and practice paternalistically embodied in the doctor was given as unproblematic (May et al. 2004). Since then, the traditional model of medical decision-making in which doctors use their knowledge, skills and judgement to make decisions on behalf of their patients has come under increasing pressure (Coulter 1997) from models such as patient-centred medicine (Stewart et al. 1995) and shared decision-making (Charles et al. 1997). Thus, doctors can no longer rely on a paternalistic model of medical practice in which the patient will act as requested because of the position of authority of the doctor, but rather a persuasive model of the relationship is increasingly perceived to be more appropriate (Scambler and Britten 2001). This implies negotiations in relation to two kinds of expertise: the authoritative general expertise of the doctor, often conceptualized as professional knowledge; and the specific experience of the patient, often conceptualized as lay beliefs (May et al. 2004). In summary, it has been suggested that: the doctor–patient relationship is changing rapidly towards a more active partnership, fostered by the increasing access to information about treatments and the consumerist trends in modern society (Elwyn et al. 1999).

Despite statements in policy documents and discussions in the academic literature, details of what partnership is and what it involves in practice are still under negotiation (Gabe et al. 2004). Moreover, Gwyn pointed to the difficulty of assessing people's preferences for involvement in consultations:

> Either patients are at ease with the consensual acceptance of power asymmetry, or else they resist it; they view doctors' attempts to involve them more comprehensively in the decision-making process either with suspicion or else as bona fide attempts by the doctor to achieve fuller patient collaboration. Between these extremities lies the mass of consultations.
>
> (2002: 74–5)

Patients may not be ready and willing to take on increased decision-making responsibilities (Coulter 1999; Calnan and Gabe 2001; Dunn 2002), preferring their doctor to make decisions for them (Makoul et al. 1995; McKinstry 2000). It is, however, questionable, given the increasing emphasis on participation in policy documentation, whether adoption of a passive role by patients is perceived to be an acceptable option, and it is therefore timely to examine patients' views on participation in consultations.

Given the increasing focus on patient involvement, participation and partnership in the consultation, as well as the difficulties of assessing patients' preferences with regard to this, this chapter draws on interview data from 53 respondents regarding their perceptions of what makes a good or a bad consultation, focusing in particular on how the views expressed relate to notions of involvement and participation. Before doing this it is first necessary to provide a brief explanation about the way in which these terms may be defined.

As pointed out in Chapter 3 by Thompson, the terms 'involvement' and 'participation' are often used synonymously without a clear understanding of the difference between them. Thompson argues that the main distinguishing feature between patient involvement and patient participation concerns the degree to which patients take part in the decision-making process. By merely describing their symptoms in the consultation, patients may be said to have some level of involvement, while the term participation connotes a degree of transfer of power from the professional to the patient in the form of increased knowledge, control and responsibility. This chapter is concerned with statements that involve the expression of opinions or a desire to take part in discussion. The encounters referenced in these statements may be characterized as moving beyond involvement, towards participation; but they do not necessarily involve two-way communication or a sharing of power on the basis of mutual respect and openness, such as could be described as full participation.

Methods

This chapter is based on an analysis of interview data that formed part of a larger study conducted between 1996 and 1998 in which patients were followed through the consultation process. The original dataset contained data from 20 doctors and 62 patients. Patients were recruited if they were consulting either for a new problem for which they expected a prescription, or wished to discuss an issue relating to a previously prescribed medicine. They were interviewed prior to their consultation, the consultation was then audio-taped and they were interviewed approximately a week after their consultation. Further details of the methods used are presented elsewhere (Stevenson et al. 2003).

In post-consultation interviews (53 in total), patients were asked to provide their opinion as to what makes a good or a bad consultation. The demographic characteristics of the patients whose interviews are discussed here are as follows: 30 were female and 23 were male, 52 were white and one was Afro-Caribbean (self-defined). Patients varied in age from three months to 84 years of age. Although patients' socio-economic status was not recorded, the practices were deliberately drawn from rural, suburban and inner city locations in two areas in England to provide a heterogeneous sample. In the case of patients under 16, consent to participate was obtained from the person accompanying the patient and the interview was conducted either directly with, or together with, the accompanying person. Ethical approval was obtained from 11 local research ethics committees.

These qualitative interviews were conducted with people who were consulting either for a new problem for which they expected a prescription, or because they wished to discuss an issue relating to a previously prescribed medicine. The focus of the interview as a whole was not participation. This chapter draws on a small part of the interview, namely the questions concerning people's views of what makes for a good consultation or a bad one. These data have been used to consider the extent to which people's positive and negative views of consultations related to notions of participation. The advantage of this is that the responses could not have been made in line with a perceived desired response as to the benefits or disadvantages of participation.

The findings are based on a detailed analysis of responses to two questions asked at the end of an interview that had focused on a particular consultation. Patients were asked to move from consideration of a specific consultation to thinking about consultations more generally. The two general questions asked were, first, 'Thinking in general, what do you think makes a good consultation with a doctor?' and as a follow-up, 'What about a bad one?' In responding, patients drew on past experiences and/or their views and opinions. The ideas generated by patients' responses are analysed in relation to the insights they provide into patients' views about participation in consultations.

Patients' judgements of 'good' and 'bad' consultations

The analyses indicated that generally the characteristics of doctors' practices in consultations viewed positively by patients were those that could be said to provide opportunities for participation. In contrast, negative experiences were associated with consultations in which opportunities for participation appeared to be blocked. Patients considered the behaviour of doctors to be key in creating an environment in which they felt it was possible to be involved. Another area of findings concerned the relationship between doctors and patients, which was also perceived to be an important factor in determining opportunities for involvement or participation. Finally, there were some dissenting voices that were not interested in involvement and participation, preferring instead to take a passive role in the consultation.

The behaviour of doctors

There appeared to be a commonly held perception of the doctor's behaviour as key in relation to the question as to what made a good or a bad consultation. This focus on doctors' behaviour is understandable given that the basis for consultations is a perceived requirement on the part of the patient for the knowledge and services available from the doctor. Moreover, consultations normally take place in the doctor's surgery, on the doctor's 'territory'.

Patients spoke positively of doctors who were considerate, understanding and interested in the problem being presented. Patients did not like to feel that they were imposing on the doctor's time. Discussion as to what makes a bad consultation focused on behaviours such as not listening, or not seeming interested in or concerned with the patient's problems:

> **Extract 1**
> When they don't seem to have the time and don't seem to have the concern you know . . . you're just another person, stick them on antibiotics, stick them out the door, they'll be alright. And they don't take the time to find out what the problem is.
>
> (P27 - male, 24)

Another respondent replied:

> **Extract 2**
> Well, obviously, a doctor that doesn't describe . . . doesn't explain things properly to you. Sort of doctor that sort of shunts you in and out in a minute.
>
> (P3 - female, 40)

There was a general recognition that doctors do not have much time. It was suggested that if a doctor does not have sufficient time on one occasion, then another appointment should be scheduled rather than rushing the consultation:

> **Extract 3**
> If he doesn't have the time, I think I would like to know . . . so that I can make another appointment.
>
> (P32 - male, 40)

It was suggested that the doctor's presence and manner should be such that patients feel able to discuss even intimate matters, thus facilitating patient participation. It was further suggested that if the patient were able to relax and feel comfortable while discussing their problems, then this would enhance the smooth running of the consultation. In terms of personal characteristics, there was a common feeling against doctors who were perceived to be abrupt, patronizing, bad-tempered or overly efficient. Patients were critical of doctors who appeared unapproachable, who made them feel uncomfortable or that they were silly to have consulted. The view expressed was that doctors, as professionals, should hold their personal feelings in check:

> **Extract 4**
> I think a doctor needs to make you feel as though you are not being silly. I know sometimes it can't be easy, because they are not always going to feel in that good a mood and I think they have to put that on one side and not make you feel uncomfortable.
>
> (P10 - female, 51)

The anxiety patients may feel before consulting was also raised by one respondent who discussed how consulting involved the fear of the unknown:

> **Extract 5**
> I think I'm not the only one who has a feeling of dread at them finding something more serious or . . . sometimes embarrassing . . . depending on what it is.
>
> (P53 - female, 48)

Much of what patients discussed involved their belief that the doctor was responsible for creating an atmosphere in which patients would feel comfortable. In practice, it was suggested doctors should give their full attention to the patient, look at the patient when they were talking and not write at the same time. Some patients focused on the example of prescribing to illustrate behaviours they disliked. They suggested that in some cases prescriptions were used as a substitute for care and were seemingly written as they walked in prior to any discussion of the presenting problem, as well as being used as a way to terminate a consultation:

> **Extract 6**
> I really don't like to see a doctor reaching for their pen and pad as they're talking to you, as though the prescription is the be all and end all of what the problem is, how it can be treated. I do think on some occasions that they don't want prescriptions but just some little . . . advice or another way of looking at it or . . . you, to be examined so that it might not be something that requires a prescription.
>
> (P53 - female, 48)

The importance of doctors' conduct in consultations was further emphasized by one respondent suggesting that feeling understood and reassured was likely to lead to a positive conclusion to the consultation:

Extract 7

Understanding, I think that's very important, sympathy . . . be empathic . . . and come out of the consultation like you feel something's been solved or . . . happy. Come out of it happy, reassured.

(P34 - female, 21)

This is in keeping with the line taken in Extract 6, that an actual treatment may not be necessary, thus highlighting the importance of the doctor's manner in the consultation. Indeed, in recounting a previous experience, another patient, in Extract 8, made a distinction between technical expertise (lines 1–2) and consultation skills (lines 3–9), indicating that technical skills alone may not necessarily be sufficient for a consultation to be judged positively:

Extract 8

Well, I had a bad one, what I considered a bad one . . . the advice was sound but the presentation of that advice was bloody awful. He never even picked his head up from the table. He just looked . . . sat at the table there and I sat there and he looked . . . and all he did was look at the table and the computer, while he was talking to me and I am thinking and I hate that . . . It wouldn't have hurt him to just turn his chair round on the side and have a few words before we started you know and then sort of make a point of looking at you when he talked to you, rather than just look at his notes . . . that is the sort I don't like. Very efficient, but very old-fashioned way, I think, of doing things.

(P9 - male, 66)

The most common and often initial response to the question as to what makes a good consultation was that the doctor listened and encouraged involvement in discussions about the presenting problem. Key to this seemed to be the feeling that the doctor was treating the patient as an individual person with their own views and opinions, as opposed to just a collection of symptoms. (This point was similarly made in Extract 1, in which a patient expressed a dislike at being treated as 'just another person'.)

Extract 9

Well, I think if he . . ., you know, the doctor listens to what you have got to say and then discusses it with you, I think that is about it, isn't it?

(P2 - female, 84)

Patients thought that it was important that doctors listened to their agendas. When discussing this, some respondents focused on the significance of the information that patients bring to the consultation:

> **Extract 10**
> The information the patient brings to the situation is important and their understanding of what is wrong, and I think you know a good doctor will try and find that out.
>
> (P21 - female, mother of child aged 3)

Thus, not only was a preference expressed for consultations in which there were opportunities for participation, it was also suggested that patient participation had a value in enhancing the consultation. Having said this, the level and type of participation sought need to fit with the patient's agenda. One patient recounted an incident in which the doctor appeared to be following his own agenda in relation to a different problem, at the expense of proper consideration of the reason for her consultation on that day. This prevented the patient from focusing on what she considered to be the problem, and presented a potential challenge to the decision to consult about that particular problem. It also suggested that the doctor's view of what was important or interesting was taking precedence over the patient's judgement of what needed to be discussed at that point in time:

Extract 11 (I = interviewer; P = patient)

I: What things do you think would make a bad consultation?

P: When you go in with one problem and the doctor starts looking through your notes and talking about another problem and that's what one of the doctors did to me not so long ago in there. Instead of taking any interest in the problem I've got, he started reading through my notes and discussing my blood and what was I doing about my blood and what was and how was it being dealt with, and this and that and the other and I came out of there so cross, the fact that you know, yes, I ended up with some sort of tablets or what have you for the problem that I went for, but I didn't honestly feel that that had been dealt with properly because he was far more interested and he literally was going back through quite a lot of my notes, um, just looking and I just, I just didn't feel that there was a need for him to be going back through my notes for other problems when I'd gone to him for something totally different that I was asking him to deal with. And that to me was wrong, and that's one of the ones I won't go and see now because I just didn't feel happy with the way he dealt with it.

(P11 - female, 43)

It is worth noting that, in this particular instance, the presenting problem was treated (lines 9–10), and the patient's account suggests her participation with respect to information about the problem was sought in the consultation (lines 6–8). However, the patient did not feel the problem for which she had consulted had been adequately dealt with, because of the focus given by the doctor to her prior and ongoing problems (lines 10–16). Thus the issue is not just about involving patients in consultations, but also involving them in a way they perceive to be appropriate.

One respondent pointed to the importance of the doctor accepting the patient's description of the symptoms as accurate. When asked to discuss what he did not like in a consultation, he responded:

Extract 12

I would think somebody who makes it obvious that they don't agree or can't accept what you are saying as factual.

(P1 - male, 69)

This comment, in common with those about doctors making patients feel uncomfortable in the consultation, details behaviours that 'block' opportunities for patient participation.

There was some discussion of the need for doctors to respect their patients, to treat them as equals and to tailor information to patients' needs and understanding:

Extract 13

It's a tall order I know but – but try – if a – if at all possible – trying to meet the patient as an equal, I think, you know, on – on sort of common ground, and I mean, historically, that's not been the case with doctors has it. Erm, a lot of doctors are very good at it now and I think some are still a bit entrenched in old ways.

(P21 - female, mother of child aged 3)

Extract 14

I think . . . a GP who is on the same wavelength, who doesn't speak down to you . . . um . . . who measures your . . . I think your intellectual ability to understand what he's saying . . . your need or otherwise for reassurance, information, . . . and tries to tailor his responses to your needs and level of understanding.

(P45 - male, 46)

The focus was on treating each patient as an individual, and tailoring consultations. It was further suggested that a possible way in which such preferences may be translated into practice was through the training doctors receive before becoming GPs. Thus, when asked what advice he would give to a young doctor training to become a GP, one patient replied as follows:

> **Extract 15**
> I think truly just to be more human than android like, not to be too . . . don't talk down to anybody, try to see them at a level that you would want to be seen yourself . . . Treat them as you'd like to be treated yourself if you were a patient.
>
> (P32 - male, 40)

However, alongside the discussion about equality and respect there was the acknowledgement that the patient is also actively seeking expert advice or treatment. Indeed, the importance of the doctor's role in providing advice, explanations and reassurance was stressed by the same patient:

> **Extract 16**
> Doctors' skills as well, the knowledge . . . obviously has to be there, and . . . to use it to reassure. The knowledge to reassure is in my opinion a very precious thing, because you can reassure somebody just by a few words ((unclear words)) than a bunch of tablets.
>
> (P32 - male, 40)

Knowledge of the patient's medical background was said to ease the flow of the consultation. A knowledgeable doctor facilitates participation, as patients then feel comfortable discussing options and acting on the advice and explanations provided. Although respondents valued having their questions answered, they also preferred doctors to admit to any gaps in their knowledge. This did not appear to adversely affect their opinion of the doctor:

> **Extract 17**
> I think they've got to be prepared, like, if, if you've got a doctor that, that's prepared to, erm, admit he doesn't know.
>
> (P13 - male, 61)

Thus, it is not just knowledge that may be seen to facilitate participation, but also trust. Trust in the doctor plays a large part, as patients expressed the need to feel that they are making decisions based on an honest exchange of information, which includes the admission of any gaps in the knowledge base.

The discussion thus far has focused on patients' preferences in relation to doctors' behaviour in the consultation. Specifically, it has considered how doctors' conduct may facilitate or block opportunities for involvement and participation. The preferences expressed illustrate an appetite for participation.

Another area of findings concerns patients' views about the doctor–patient relationship.

The relationship between doctors and patients

Patients stressed the importance of having a relationship with the doctor in which they felt comfortable expressing their thoughts and opinions. For the most part, the doctor was perceived to be responsible for creating and maintaining the relationship. There were also suggestions that patients should take responsibility for acting if the relationship does not appear to be working. There was some disagreement about the need to maintain a professional distance in the relationship with their doctor. Some respondents talked of being able to chat to their doctor as if they were a friend:

> **Extract 18**
> You feel like you're going in and talking to a friend . . . he is very easy to talk to.
>
> (P32 - male, 40)

Others commented that a certain distance was necessary, and drew a distinction between a cordial versus a friendly relationship:

> **Extract 19**
> I think it's probably not healthy to develop an over-friendly relationship with a doctor . . . I don't think professionally it would make it as easy for him to be dispassionate . . . it is better to be on cordial than on friendly terms, I think.
>
> (P18 - male, 46)

In line with most of the comments made by patients in the interviews, the discussion thus far has focused on the suggestion that the doctor's behaviour is the crucial factor in the production of what were judged to be good consultations, and in particular for creating the conditions that make participation possible. However, some patients suggested that the onus should be on patients themselves to facilitate their participation in the consultation. For example, some patients said they had a responsibility to articulate their problems clearly, to enable the doctor to work to the best of their ability:

> **Extract 20**
> I think that if the communication is there, provided you tell the doctor everything and answer all his questions straightforwardly, quite clearly he can give you his best advice, but if you come away and if I

> come away and think, 'Gosh, I should have told him that'. . . it's my fault, not his.
>
> (P40 - male, 59)

This suggests a definite role, and even a responsibility relating to participation, on the part of the patient. Some also said that patients should not be too demanding, suggesting that they should exercise moderation in their expectations of consultations:

> **Extract 21**
>
> I don't think I would go in with an attitude, y'know, I want the best and I've got to have this and that, I think that wouldn't help, y'know, but go in as yourself.
>
> (P8 - female, 67)

Moving on from this, the comments of one respondent in particular presented the consultation as a joint endeavour between doctors and patients, based on respect for each other's roles, with a sharing of responsibility for the final outcome:

> **Extract 22**
>
> It's a two-way thing and I think a lot of people believe it is one-way . . . it is not a cat and mouse game. It is communication.
>
> (P5 - female, 53)

This, and Extract 23, present the relationship as a communication partnership between the doctor and the patient, much as has been suggested in the policy documentation and academic literature over the past 10 years:

> **Extract 23**
>
> To me a bad consultation is where the art of communication has broken down somewhere along the line. Whether intentionally on the patient's part or because the GP has got a preconceived idea.
>
> (P5 - female, 53)

As has been illustrated, most of the behaviours that respondents associated with a 'good' consultation may be said in some way to enhance the possibility of patient participation in the consultation. There were, however, some dissenting voices that expressed a preference for consultations in which their involvement was minimal.

Dissenting voices

In contrast to the majority of respondents who talked of the importance of behaviours that may be seen as facilitating participation, such as listening and taking account of the patient's viewpoint, and involving patients in discussions about their problems, there were dissenting voices, with some patients presenting a more passive model in which the doctor's skills in diagnosis and treatment were viewed to be of major importance. Thus, it was suggested that the key to a good consultation was that the doctor should:

Extract 24

Find out what's wrong with you and give you what you need.

(P38 - female, 31)

This emphasises the importance of the doctor getting it right technically; there was no associated discussion of the importance of the participation or involvement of the patient. Thus, when judging the merits of consultations, patients may not always perceive behaviours that facilitate opportunities for participation to be of prime importance.

Despite the fact that consultations in which the patient perspective was ignored were generally presented negatively, one respondent was critical of the doctor asking her what she thought was wrong, suggesting this was indicative of a lack of knowledge on the part of the doctor, as opposed to a desire for her input:

Extract 25 (I = interviewer; P = patient)

P: Sometimes I've had said to me, what do you think is the matter? Well, if I knew what was the matter, I wouldn't have been there in the first place . . . I feel that's for her to find out, not me particularly.

I: What do you think leads doctors to ask that question?

P: Perhaps when they don't really know themselves.

(P38 - female, 51)

This demonstrates the danger of a blanket policy that patients should be involved in consultations. The presentation of the consultation as a joint endeavour can be juxtaposed against comments from patients who did not feel it was necessary for them to contribute and, indeed, were critical of the opportunity to do so. Thus, it is impossible to create a 'blueprint' or model for how consultations should be conducted that would be acceptable to all in all circumstances. This supports the point made in Chapter 3 by Thompson that the desire for involvement needs to be optional and varies according to the context of the consultation and probably over time as well.

There was, however, an awareness of changes in wider society that have had an impact on the consultation and its operation at the micro level. It was suggested that doctors were becoming more like service providers and patients more like customers, thus requiring a change in the way in which doctors present themselves:

Extract 26

We're getting more into a situation where the doctor is the service provider and the people that come to see him are the customers . . . and consequently that requires a change in the way that they present themselves.

(P31 - male, 34)

Another change in society that is likely to have had an impact on the relationship between doctors and patients is the availability of information about a range of issues, including health:

Extract 27

We've all read enough, in various magazines if nothing else, to know a certain amount about things.

(P33 - female, 40)

Thus, in general a traditional model of the doctor–patient relationship, in which the doctor makes decisions solely on the basis of their own knowledge, is likely to be unacceptable.

Summary of findings

Generally patients were positive about consultations in which there were opportunities for participation, and negative about consultations in which opportunities for participation appeared to be blocked. The doctor's behaviour was perceived to be crucial in creating the conditions that make participation possible. There was only limited discussion of the responsibilities of patients in the consultation and of shared responsibilities.

Patients disliked doctors who did not appear to listen or explain, did not seem interested or concerned and made them feel that they were imposing on the doctor's time (Extracts 1, 2, 3). They stressed the need to feel comfortable in the consultation (Extract 4), highlighting the anxiety that is often associated with consulting (Extract 5). Indeed, it was suggested that the doctor's conduct in the consultation might be judged to be of greater importance in terms of the outcome than a prescription (Extracts 6, 7 and 8). This corroborates the work of Mercer and colleagues in emphasizing the importance of empathy shown by the practitioner (Mercer and Reynolds 2002; Mercer et al. 2002).

Patients liked to be listened to and encouraged to take part (Extract 9), and the patient's perspective was judged to be important (Extract 10). Having said this, patients should be involved in a way that they perceive to be appropriate. The importance of the way in which patient's views are received was stressed (Extract 12), with a number of comments expressing a desire for doctors to respect patients and their contributions (Extracts 12, 13, 14, 15). Yet, comments about the need to respect the patient were in no way seen to detract from the importance of the doctor's skills and knowledge in reassuring patients (Extract 16). A preference was also expressed for doctors to admit to any gaps in their knowledge (Extract 17).

Differing views were expressed concerning the ideal type of relationship between doctors and patients. Some people talked of being able to chat to their doctor as if they were a friend (Extract 18), while others felt there should be some distance observed (Extract 19). It was suggested that patients had a responsibility to present their problems clearly (Extract 20) and should be moderate in their expectations (Extract 21). One patient in particular presented the consultation as a joint endeavour, with a shared responsibility for the final outcome (Extracts 22 and 23).

Finally, some patients presented the patient's role as passive (Extracts 24 and 25), with no discussion of involvement or participation. The idea that changes in society means that doctors may now be seen as service providers (Extract 26) was raised, and comments were made concerning the availability of information about health (Extract 27). These points remind us of the societal context within which preferences for involvement or participation should be considered.

Discussion

Patients generally wanted the opportunity to express their thoughts and opinions in the consultation. A wide range of preferences were expressed; from working in partnership with the doctor, through to being a passive recipient of medical care. This fits with the notion of activists and non-activists as outlined in Chapter 3 by Thompson. As this was a qualitative study, no attempt was made to quantify the expressed preferences. In McKinstry's (2000) sample, the majority of respondents preferred a directed style rather than a shared one, but he did not investigate a wider range of preferences. His work suggests that preferences are influenced by the type of problem, patient's age, smoking status, and social class, but not their gender. Thompson's (Chapter 3, this volume) encapsulation of patient involvement as a complex, multi-faceted, dynamic concept fits with the range of ways in which people explored their preferences in relation to involvement in the consultation. Specifically, Thompson's conclusions support the idea that patients should be involved in consultations in whichever ways they perceive to be appropriate. This highlights the potential practical problem of trying to tailor consultations: not just to each individual, but also to each individual on each occasion that they consult.

Policy documents and the academic literature in this area suggest that patients should be moving towards the role of active participants in consultations. However, these data suggest that people do not expect or wish for more than limited involvement, as opposed to participation in the sense of partnership. If patients themselves do not perceive partnership as an option, or, as these data suggest, do not even desire it, then it is unlikely to happen. The crux of the problem may lie in patients' views of their relationship with their doctor. These data suggest that rather than patients viewing themselves as partners in the consultation, they perceived doctor's behaviour to be pivotal in setting the tone of the consultation, and in facilitating or blocking opportunities for patient participation. Patients generally only perceived themselves to have responsibilities (for example, taking steps to change their practitioner) if the relationship appeared problematic. Similarly, Kraetschmer et al. (2004) found that patients who expressed a desire for an autonomous role in decisions about medical treatment were those who had lower trust in their providers. Thus, although there were comments suggesting an awareness of changes in society and thus potentially in the conduct of doctors in consultations, as well as an acknowledgement of the availability of information from outside of the consultation, in general, the view held appeared to be, in line with Gwyn's (2002) work, that the majority of consultations lie between a partnership model and one in which patients are passive recipients of medical care.

Some respondents spoke in abstract terms about what they thought were good or bad elements in consultations. In most cases, however, the questions were answered in relation to specific experiences. The data may therefore be seen to be largely limited by the actual consultation experiences of respondents. Interestingly some people even felt unable to respond, as they felt their experience was insufficient.

The study from which the data originated was conducted between 1996 and 1998. The data provide a useful insight into what people thought was good and bad about consultations (and see the Educational Supplement, p. 204, for suggestions for further discussion and data collection on this theme). Arguably, if the same data were collected today, it might contain a greater number, and more diverse, references to participation, given the continuing agenda of increasing patient involvement in the NHS.

Conclusion

Respondents were generally positive about consultations in which they felt the doctor created an atmosphere that promoted involvement. Conversely, negative comments were made about doctors' behaviours that were thought to block opportunities for involvement or participation. The extent to which people appeared to wish to participate was generally at the level of being listened to and being given the time to put their viewpoint across, as well as having things explained and discussed. This is concordant with some of the views expressed regarding notions of involvement in Chapter 3 (Thompson). In the study outlined in this chapter, only one respondent talked about doctors and patients having joint responsibility in the consultation, and only two discussed how doctors should try to treat patients as equals and as they would like to be treated themselves. Thus, crucially, although the data suggest that respondents favoured behaviours that may be judged to enable participation, there was little discussion of preferences for, or experiences of, participative consultation styles in which patients might be 'active partners'. In summary, the interactions described could not accurately be characterized as 'meetings between experts' (Tuckett et al. 1985).

The data provide useful insights into the extent to which patients' views of what makes a good consultation include a preference for behaviours, in particular on the part of the doctor, that facilitate the opportunity to participate, and a dislike for behaviours that appear to block participation. Having said this, the level of participation suggested in these data is not generally suggestive of a relationship in which patients are active partners in care, as is outlined in recent policy documents and the academic literature. This could be due to the age of the data, but is arguably more likely to be a product of another salient aspect of these data; namely, that the responsibility for presenting opportunities for participation and conversely for blocking them was seen to rest with the doctor. With the exception of one patient, there seemed to be little appetite for active partnership. Thus, it may be concluded that respondents generally conceived of consultations as interactions in which, although both parties may have expertise, the influence to decide how that expertise is used rests with the doctor. Therefore, the data may be seen to illustrate how patients do not expect or wish for more than limited involvement, as opposed to participation in the sense of partnership.

Acknowledgements

The research project was funded as part of the Department of Health prescribing research initiative. The views expressed in this chapter are those of the author and not the Department of Health. The research team comprised Nick Barber, Colin Bradley, Nicky Britten, Christine Barry and Fiona Stevenson. A version of this work was presented to the London Medical Sociology Group. The author is grateful for the lively discussion and incisive comments received.

Recommendations: summary

- There is no single preferred way of involving patients in consultations.
- Each consultation is unique and requires an individualized approach.
- Patients may expect professionals to set the tone for the consultation.

5 A feeling of equality

Some interactional features that build rapport and mutuality in a therapeutic encounter

John Chatwin, Sarah Collins, Ian Watt and Rowena Field

Commentary

Continuing the theme begun in Chapter 4, of professionals' responsibility for making patients feel at ease and thus enabling their participation, this chapter documents some consultation practices of health professionals through which patients' participation may be promoted.

The starting point is the study of interaction in consultations, using conversation analysis (CA). Along with Chapters 6, 7 and 8, the presented examples and accompanying descriptions not only provide a clear demonstration of what CA is and how it works but also illustrate the potential of this approach to explore questions relating to patients' participation.

This chapter extends the arena for studying participation beyond the general practice consultation (the focus of the interviews presented in Chapter 4). Detailed reference is made to the opening of one consultation which takes place in a homoeopathic hospital which integrates complementary and orthodox medical care. This case study is supplemented by ethnographic observations, interviews with health professionals and extracts from a themed discussion between a homoeopath and a general practitioner, providing a complement to the views of patients as presented in Chapters 3 and 4.

The particular dimensions of the health care consultation explored here are mutuality, equality, rapport and empathy. The analysis identifies some qualitative features of the opening phase which help to create a feeling of equality and which thereby invite the patient's participation. The building of mutuality (in this case, through discussion about the video camera's presence, deciding on address terms, joking, and reading aloud the GP referral letter) provides a resource through which the patient is familiarized with, and begins to participate in, the holistic approach.

The particular consultation presented here is one in which the patient is new to homoeopathy. The new experience of this first homoeopathic encounter exposes some of those often hidden and taken-for-granted aspects of the consultation, and articulates these aspects in ways which invite the patient to become involved.

Introduction

Medical encounters are frequently regarded as having a potentially therapeutic value in their own right, as well as the potential for being anti-therapeutic (see, for example, Elwyn and Gwyn 1999; Reilly 2001). At a basic level, interactions between patients and practitioners have been shown to have a direct impact not just on factors such as the degree to which a person feels satisfied with the therapeutic relationship (Drew et al. 2001; Little et al. 2001; Hall et al. 2002; Schofield et al. 2003), or on the level of commitment that they are willing to invest in their treatment, but also on health-related outcomes (Greenfield et al. 1988; Stewart 1995). Frankel and West (1991), for example, outlined how patients are more likely to follow treatment recommendations if they feel they have been involved in discussion about the planned treatment (and see Rost et al. 1989; Squier 1990).

Despite awareness of the potential benefits of patient involvement, it has been reported that while involvement in decisions about when to seek professional help, who to consult, whether to continue with recommended treatment programmes, and so on, is relatively common, involvement in decisions about matters *within* the consultation, such as treatment prescriptions, is far less actively sought (Entwistle et al. 1998). A number of interventions have been developed with the aim of improving the level at which patients can actively participate in such decisions (see Chapter 1). Health professionals are increasingly incorporating inclusive concepts such as 'concordance' (see Dickinson et al. 1999; Lask 2002), or are adopting more holistic approaches such as 'narrative-based medicine' (Silverman 1987; Elwyn and Gwyn 1999; Greenhalgh and Hurwitz 1999; Launer 1999), in pursuit of a more rounded contextualization of individual patients and not just an understanding of their diseases.

This spirit of incorporation that is inspiring a significant number of health care professionals (Tovey 1997; Jump et al. 1998; Botting and Cook 2000) may have something to do with regaining elements in medicine that are perceived as being 'lost' or neglected (Hunter 1991), that is, those humanistic elements that may be obscured by the complexity of medical technology and the pace of modern consultations, but which can provide depth and richness to the therapeutic process. Research into patient motivation has suggested that much of the appeal of complementary medicine lies in patients' perceptions that the consultations will embody qualities that have somehow become attenuated in conventional medicine (Thomas et al. 1991; Vincent and Furnham 1996; Chatwin and Collins 2002).

As indicated in Chapter 1, there is a significant paucity of research indicating how behavioural approaches that engender holism and patient participation are actually enacted within discrete consultation environments. Much of what is to be gained from patient participation (more equality in the therapeutic encounter, increased involvement for patients in decisions about their treatment, and so on) is often viewed as integral to complementary medicine approaches. In many forms of complementary medicine, these more active involvement opportunities for patients, through the incorporation of more egalitarian or 'holistic' elements into the consultation process, are a key feature, but little attention has been paid to the details of the form these opportunities take, or to how they can be developed and evaluated (House of Lords 2000).

For the study on which this chapter is based (see Acknowledgement to this chapter), over 40 homoeopathic consultations (in private practice, general practice and hospital settings), were recorded alongside orthodox medical consultations (in family planning, diabetes in general practice, cancer genetics, and cancer of the head or neck). Interviews were also conducted with all participating health professionals and patients, about their views and experiences of patient participation in consultations.

Homoeopathy is currently the second most widely used form of medicine in the world – Chinese medicine is first, herbalism is third, and conventional medicine is fourth (Chappell 1999). From an interactional perspective, in homoeopathy the development or maintenance of a person's commitment to the healing process, and the reflexive role of the practitioner, hold a particular relevance in therapeutic terms; the stimulation of the patient's natural healing abilities underpin the treatment process. This is not only because of the direct humanistic impact of emotional and intellectual alliances between a patient and practitioner, but also because the art of prescribing the ultra-dilute remedies that the system utilizes relies on the interpretation of many subtle psychological, non-verbal and narrative cues – cues that are, by implication, more accessible if there is a good interactional connection.

In this chapter we will outline some of the contextual and interactional motifs that appear to be significant in generating feelings of equality and mutuality. In order to do so, we will make specific and detailed reference to the opening sequences of one therapeutic encounter, recorded in an NHS homoeopathic hospital that integrates conventional with complementary forms of medicine. The focus will be on the processes of communication in the consultation, and how these engender participation, and on the identification of features and practices that may be applied to any form of health care encounter. In-depth investigation of processes of interaction in consultations has the potential to inform a variety of health care settings and types of consultation, while at the same time identifying features that may be considered distinctive of a particular professional discipline, health care specialty, or approach.

Prior to the presentation of a single case, to illuminate features that promote a feeling of equality, we will consider the effects of the therapeutic environment, focusing on ways in which features of the environment influence the arena for patients' participation and the opportunities made available for participation. This first part of the chapter is based largely on ethnographic observational data from hospital and general practice settings, interviews with health care professionals collected as part of a project exploring patient participation in decision-making (see the Acknowledgement to this chapter; Entwistle et al. 2004; Farrell 2004), and longer narrative fragments taken from a themed discussion between a homoeopath and a general practitioner, recorded specifically to inform this chapter.

In the second part of the chapter we shift from the broad contextualization provided by the ethnographic data to focus on the interactional details of a real consultation. Here, we employ conversation analysis to describe the ways in which mutuality, and states such as empathy and rapport, are generated by the doctor, and how these invite the patient's active contribution (and preparatory or follow-up exercises are provided in the Educational Supplement, see pp. 205–7).

Where encounters take place

The environments in which medical encounters of any kind take place are obviously important and have their effect on a patient's participation (for example, see the Afterword to this book). For some people, even the smell of a hospital can induce panic. At a less extreme level, the kinds of impressions and interactions to which people are exposed when they visit a health professional all help to generate a particular frame of reference. The physical environment has been reported to have a significant influence on patients' experiences of, and feelings about, the care they receive (Mercer and Reilly 2004). The places where homoeopaths work tend to be significantly different from those of conventional practitioners; their surgeries rarely have the 'medical' atmosphere of hospitals or doctors' practices, and are generally free of the bureaucratic structures that can reinforce an institutional separation between a doctor and a patient.

'Enhancing the Healing Environment' (Kings Fund 2006) is an England-based programme which has demonstrated the difference environment can make to the healing capacity of hospitals. Initiatives have included the creation of more normal spaces within the hospital environment, and room and corridor designs that safeguard patient confidentiality and dignity, that ensure protected therapeutic time, and that have motivated patients to take the initiative in approaching health professionals and to select where they spend their time and who they talk with while in hospital. The Glasgow Homoeopathic Hospital in Scotland has been purpose-built, to be, as traditionally intended for all hospitals, 'places of rest and beauty that would enhance human healing' (Glasgow Homoeopathic Hospital 2006).

Doctors working within conventional medicine are more likely to face the restrictions of working within a large public health service. For example, in the hospital head and neck cancer clinics visited during our research, health professionals and patients spoke of the difficulties and implications of this highly public encounter for patients: meeting 'a sea of faces'; 'the gaggle' in the waiting room; the crowdedness and the chaos on particularly busy afternoons. As one surgeon reported:

> **Extract 1**
> I think a lot of them are probably, first of all, totally overwhelmed by what they've just heard. Completely mind-boggled. Secondly, I think they're probably quite intimidated, by me, and the room, and the hangers-on, and the whole thing.
>
> (Interview, ENT surgeon, D2–102)

The speech and language therapist in the same clinic said:

> **Extract 2**
> I do think it's dreadful for some patients when they walk into that clinic room with [the surgeon] and five other people, that must be dreadful and not for everyone to be introduced. And for people to walk in and out of the clinic room when they are discussing treatment options. I don't think that's an ideal way to be comfortable while you're thinking about surgical and treatment options . . . so the environment I think could be better.
>
> (Interview, Speech and language therapist, A-103)

The surgeon detailed how, on the ward, various disruptions in the environment made it hard to talk without interruption:

> **Extract 3**
> There's other patients being taken off to theatre. There's sometimes an awkward patient sitting in the bed next to you who's making a lot of noise. Even if you managed to get an isolated room, you've got people coming in and out. I think it's a rather disruptive . . . The other thing, particularly on the modern wards is, I'm quite sure that if I was in hospital with any ENT ailment other than cancer I'd be bored to

tears. And if someone was talking about some horrendous operation behind the curtains I'd be, very aware of it and listening in. So it's not really very – a nice environment, for the patient who then has to go and stay in the ward and look the other people in the eye and to feel you know, 'you know all about what I've just been told'.

(Interview, ENT surgeon, D2-102)

He reported how the ward environment altered the way he spoke:

Extract 4

You don't tend to be too gruesome. You don't tend to talk about prognosis or anything like that. I tend to talk in – *Reader's Digest*-type terms about operations and whether they're complicated or easy. I don't tend to go into detail.

(Interview, ENT surgeon, D2-102)

And he contrasted this with his consultations with patients in the clinic:

Extract 5

You do know in the clinic setting that you're not going to have – suddenly – some completely diverting catastrophe happening in the room. So you know you've got 15 minutes. You know it's going to be relatively quiet, and you can get on with it, without any diversions.

(Interview, ENT surgeon, D2-102)

In the discussion recorded for the purposes of developing the themes of this chapter, we asked a GP and a homoeopath to each comment on their experiences and use of environmental features in their consultations with patients. The GP commented:

Extract 6

I think there probably is quite a lot of thought in general practice about making it a comfortable environment. Until relatively recently at least this contrasts quite sharply with hospitals, I mean [there are lots of] examples of hospitals where the environment is awful and consulting rooms are horrible and the waiting rooms are horrible and that's partly to do with the resources of the NHS but in part it's also I think down to a lack of imagination of the people running the hospitals, although this is starting to change . . . We're aware of the effects physical environment can have but it's still a health centre, so there's a degree of a clinical feel around it but we try and keep that to a minimum, you know, there's plants around, we do think about colours. But having said that there are some gimmicks, it's a surgery, not someone's home.

(GP, themed discussion)

In purely practical terms, the homoeopathic patient is likely to engage with the environment where their treatment takes place in a different way. They will be, for example, unlikely to encounter long delays in crowded and impersonal waiting rooms, or have the feeling that they are in a place where time is always at a premium. Many homoeopaths have their surgeries in their homes and patients will routinely find themselves in surroundings that are consciously designed to be calm and relaxing – environments that exhibit a particularly holistic '*rhetoric of legitimisation*' (Ball 1967). In the homoeopathic arena, this rhetoric (which includes everything from visual and audio cues to symbols and scents) is used overtly as a means of generating an interactional space that, while 'professional', may be conspicuously different from conventional medical environments:

Extract 7

I work from home and from a clinic. The home is where you're relaxed. I mean, at home, it has its own drawbacks because it's not a specific healing space if you like, but it is part of a living room, so there are the things of life around. The clinic I work from, that is a clinic space [but] a lot of thought has gone into the lighting and arrangements of bookcases and what sort of books, fish tanks and literature for people to read and the sort of chairs for them to sit in the waiting area. It's all important. At home, I don't have a desk in the living room, it's just, you know, things on my knees and it's all very relaxed. I know some people just feel happier in a more formal setting, [for] other people it's like a sigh of relief that it's just like the interior of someone's home.

(Homoeopath, themed discussion)

One aspect of environment concerns how entry into any consultation is entangled within a psychological and social framework of preconceptions, past experiences, and other encounters. No medical encounter occurs in isolation, and in the case of consultations involving homoeopathic approaches, both patient and practitioner often bring with them ingrained ideas of the look and feel of other, often more traditional medical consultations, and this naturally colours the way in which they view what takes place as their interactions together unfold. For the new homoeopathic patient, the events leading up to and including the first consultation are important. They are likely to engender feelings of novelty and strangeness; perhaps, even, a vague sense of unease at stepping outside the socially sanctioned world of orthodox medicine. For some people, seeking out a more holistic approach can even be seen as a reflection of deeper subconscious processes. It may, as one homoeopath in our study suggested, reflect the first stirrings of a kind of psychological or even spiritual self-development, of acknowledging that there are other perspectives on health and scientific reality. People who try holistic medicine may find that the experience represents something more than simply going to a 'different kind of doctor', even if at a conscious level this is all they are doing. As with counselling or psychotherapy, the knock-on effects of the homoeopathic process with its emphasis on deeper empathetic connections can have a profound impact on a person's outlook and persona, and again, maybe at a subconscious level, this is what some people are seeking.

In a first health care encounter in an unfamiliar environment, a patient may initially be highly sensitive to the entire bundle of interactions and impressions that surround the experience. There may be particular expectations, perhaps having heard stories of how 'different', or 'not like going to the doctor', the experience will be. If genuine trust and rapport are to be built up as the therapeutic relationship develops, everything the patient encounters and assimilates as their socialization proceeds ideally needs to be synchronized with holistic principles so that discordant elements are reduced to a minimum.

A therapeutic encounter in a hospital setting

The interaction environments that border the consultation embody, as discussed above, a kind of preparatory groundwork. Once the consultation proper begins, the practitioner and patient can start to make more concrete inroads into developing a working relationship that is rich in mutuality, and that foregrounds opportunities for the patient to contribute and participate. By mutuality, we mean forms of equality which are made manifest in interaction by, for example, a greeting which positions both participants similarly (such as 'Hello, Dr Smith, how are you?' and the return 'Hello, Mr Brown, I'm fine, thank you, how are you?'), or a reference (as will be seen below) to the researcher's video camera in the consultation that invites both participants equally to voice any concern about its presence. For a conceptual overview of mutuality and related concepts, as employed in the study of dialogue, see Graumann (1995). For studies of empathy and related concepts in health care settings, see Reynolds (2000); Branch et al. (2001); Mercer et al. (2002); Rudebeck (2002).

In order to illustrate some ways in which this process may be managed, we will now concentrate on the opening minutes of a consultation involving a patient new to the homoeopathic hospital, and unfamiliar with the rhythms and routines of holistic medicine. This encounter has been chosen for two reasons. First, this particular practitioner was actively interested in developing deep interactional connections within his consultations. The encounter may therefore be something of a 'showcase' of good practice, regarding the processes of patient participation. Second, this consultation represents an integrative, holistic approach, which combines orthodox and complementary medicine and which employs elements of each in the patient's care. Thus, the data from this single case are presented to illustrate the potential of employing various details of interaction, and of drawing on environmental influences, in order to enhance a patient's participation.

In this type of first-time consultation, interactional strategies for the generation of mutuality are likely to be close to the surface because, as with any medical encounter, the initial 'feel' that a patient gets from a practitioner (and vice versa), represents an important datum upon which subsequent contacts are founded. If there are serious misalignments at this early stage of the relationship, a good deal of effort will be required later on to repair them – effort that would obviously be better directed towards the therapeutic process itself. In extreme cases, misalignments at this baseline level prove unrecoverable. One homoeopathic patient we were able to interview, for example, described how it was interactional misalignments during an initial consultation that made her decide not to return for a second time. It can be assumed therefore, that this is a sensitive point in the consultation sequence (especially as the patient may have had a long wait for a referral, or perhaps be paying for the consultation). To some extent, then, the practitioner is likely to be capitalizing on every means available to ensure that the image that they project will be the most efficacious in aligning them with the patient on as many levels as possible.

In line with this, the consultation extract (Extract 8) is an illustration of how, in the hands of an experienced practitioner, virtually any aspect of interaction with the patient may be utilized in the generation of mutuality, and may consequently create a host of opportunities for the patient's participation. The patient here had been referred to this practitioner (a medically qualified homoeopathic doctor) by his GP, after being on a waiting list for some months. The extract covers the first four minutes or so of the consultation. Just prior to the beginning of the transcript the practitioner met the patient in the surgery waiting area and some informal talk had taken place. The practitioner had checked, for example, that the patient was still happy for the researcher to video-record the encounter. The talk begins as both parties are seated in the consultation room:

Extract 8 (D = doctor; P = patient)

```
D:  . . . so as I say (0.2) if (.) either of us (0.3) want
    that off (0.4) or afterwards chucked
    (0.5)
P:  Right
D:  We- either of us must feel free to say that
P:  H-hm
    (.)
D:  Yea? (0.3) okay (0.5) ah my name's Alan Benway
    (0.3)
P:  Right
```

```
        (0.3)
    D:  So I-I'm (0.2)·hh (0.5) some-some patients are
        comfortable just to call me Alan or Doctor Alan,
        or Doctor Benway (0.2) whatever's natural
        (0.4)
    P:  W'll- what do you (0.3) prefe[r
    D:                                   [Ye- (.) wh- you just
        wh- any way you want
    P:  ^Wh-[h·-hu-[hu-hu
    D:      [Okay  [what-what - what do you like to be
        called w[h-
    P:          [Er- (0.2)Billy
    D:  Billy (0.4) okay thank-s: Billy
        (0.5)
    P:  °Er:° (0.4) my wife's got various names for
        me[°(though)°
    D:    [^KH·<ha-ha> °picked up a pen that doesn't
        work - there it is° (0.2) °I bet you she does°
        ^k-h·-hu (0.7) let me just (.) re-read the
        letter that doctor smith wrote
        (0.2)
    P:  Right
    D:  If I could (0.3) erm ((D reads letter))
        (21.0)
    D:  tk-·h actually maybe I could read you the
        letter out
        (0.3)
    P:  Aie=
    D:  =That will let you know what I know (0.3) [then we=
    P:                                            [Right
    D:  =can kick off on the story ·hh
        ((D reads aloud from referral letter))
        . . wonder if you could have a look at this
        gentleman who has asked for a referral to the
        hospital . . .
        ((D continues reading aloud for approx 1 minute))
    D:  . . the doctor also tells me that you suffered
        from proctitus
    P:  H-hm
        (0.7)
    D:  ((Reading aloud)) 'which can f:- range from mildly
        inconvenient to totally disabling'
        (0.3)
```

P: That ws:- (0.7) when you asked me about lunch
(0.5)
D: Okay
P: ((unclear))
D: Okay ((reading aloud)) *'we seem to have reached a*
point where we've exhausted the treatments for
urticaria that we've offered, and he wondered about
homoeopathy. I'd be interested to know if you feel
that this sort of thing can be helped.'
(0.7)
P: °H-hm°
D: So that's what I- that's th- that's what I
know so far so ·hh you kick off at any point
you want really with the [story
P: [W'll that-that's - that's
more or less it . . .

(Video-recorded consultation in homoeopathy, AB-XS-1)

Even in this relatively short extract, three distinct sequential activities or phases display a directly mutualistic function, and thus encourage and promote the patient's participation. Broadly, these are:

1. The sequence of talk about the video at the start of the interaction (lines 1–6), where the practitioner re-checks that both he and the patient ('either of us', line 1 and line 5) are happy to be videoed.
2. The naming sequence (lines 8–26), in which there is some discussion about names, and what the practitioner and patient should call each other, and at the end of which there is overt development of a rapport and a point of contact (line 25).
3. An instance of 'deeper socialization' (lines 42–69) in which the practitioner reads aloud from the patient's referral letter.

We now consider each of these sequences in turn.

Talk about the video

We have chosen to include the apparently superfluous sequence that occurs at the very beginning of the consultation (lines 1–6). Ordinarily, this kind of transitional talk would probably not be of interest. It might even, because of its subject matter (the presence of the recording equipment, set up by the researcher before he left the room) be treated as something to ignore because it detracts from the 'naturalness' of the interaction. In the context of the mutuality that we are mapping, however, the way in which this talk is undertaken plays a significant role in grounding the subsequent interaction. It occurs as a kind of bridge between the informal talk that occurred on the way to the consultation room, and the 'formal' beginning of the consultation (line 8). The practitioner is able to utilize its apparently tangential topicality to begin to acclimatize the patient into the more overt mutuality of his holistic approach. Although reference to the camera is treated as a sub-issue, separate from the 'real' business of the consultation (the doctor's 'okay' on line 8 and the following 0.5 second pause that delineate the end of the topic), the way in which the doctor frames his comments conveys to the patient a sense that issues of privacy and mutual respect really are of genuine concern. We are not suggesting that this kind of activity would not occur in other medical settings but pointing out that, in this particular case, the doctor chooses to capitalize on the video camera's presence as a means of conveying mutuality. He knows that the patient has given permission for the camera to be present and could simply have indicated where it was, or even, as in the case of other health professionals whose consultations we recorded, make no reference to it whatsoever. On line 1, however, when the doctor says: '. . . so as I say if either of us want that off or afterwards chucked', he is doing something more than simply checking with the patient that the camera is still acceptable, because he is revisiting the topic within a more formal contextual frame. The two parties are no longer chatting informally in the corridor, but are now seated in the consultation room where their respective roles as patient and practitioner are more defined. For the patient at least, this is likely to imbue anything that is said from this point with greater significance. Similarly, when the doctor speaks about the camera, he is in effect drawing attention to the fact that it is recording what is being said at that moment, and this further serves to reinforce the gravity of his comments. He treats them as worthy of being recorded, of becoming part of their interaction. By utilizing this initial transitional period when the patient is likely to be highly sensitive to the newness of the encounter, the doctor begins to set a precedent for the subsequent interaction without overtly appearing to do so – the apparently 'administrative' nature of the sequence effectively masks the underlying message that it generates.

Opportunities to interact with patients in an informal pre-consultation setting have their practical therapeutic uses too. Because (as made explicit in the homoeopathic model, but also evident in other types of consultation), every aspect of the patient's behaviour may prove to be diagnostically relevant, the opportunity to observe them interacting outside (or at least tangentially to) their patient role is valuable; how they hold themselves as they move, how they talk and act when they feel that they are not under the professional's gaze, and so on. Informal pre-consultation activities, such as the small talk that takes place as the patient and practitioner settle down, can also perform the function of making the transition to the actual homoeopathic interaction more diffuse; elements of mutuality that surface during the pre-consultation interaction can be carried over into the consultation itself, making the activity boundary less abruptly defined (and see Chapter 8).

A further sub-textual function that may be attributed to this sequence is that the practitioner is able to communicate the feeling that to a certain extent, both he and the patient have a joint responsibility for what transpires, and that both have an active role to play. The doctor's language, for example, is collaborative; rather than saying 'if you want the camera off . . .', he says 'if either of us . . .' (line 1). Similarly, he says 'We . . . must feel free to say that', rather than 'You must feel free . . .' (line 5). The use of 'we' emphasizes mutuality by aligning the patient with himself, casting doctor and patient as equal under the alien gaze of the camera. It is as if the doctor deliberately picks on the camera's intrusive and mechanical presence to emphasize the value of the human connection he wishes to create; the camera is referred to as 'that' (line 1), and its tapes can be '. . . afterwards chucked' (line 2). Similarly, by acknowledging that it is not only the patient who may wish the camera to be turned off, but also himself, the doctor communicates a subtle sense of vulnerability which may further help to equalize the interactional dynamics of the developing relationship.

The naming sequence

The termination of the talk about the camera is indicated in line 8, with the doctor's 'Yea?', followed by 'okay', and this launches the transition to the start of the consultation proper. Following a 0.5 second pause, the doctor introduces himself: '. . . ah my name's Alan Benway' (line 8). The following talk (from lines 9 to 26) relate to the business of introductions. As with the earlier talk about the video, however, this activity also frames a subtext that continues to draw the patient into regarding the relationship with this doctor as subtly different from other medical relationships he may be used to. The fact that the doctor first gives his name without the prefix 'doctor' immediately implies a degree of informality and distances him from the medical associations that the more formal title obviously engenders. What may be more significant, however, is that in an extended turn following the patient's 'Right' (line 10), he goes on to offer a number of alternative naming options that are progressively more formal: 'Alan', 'Doctor Alan', and 'Doctor Benway'. This indicates that the doctor is wary of forcing informality on the patient; not everyone will feel at ease calling their doctor by his first name, especially at this early stage in the relationship. At the beginning of this turn too (line 12), the doctor says: 'some patients are comfortable just to call me . . .'. By invoking the acts of previous patients, and effectively sanctioning them, he implies that any choice this patient makes will be similarly sanctioned. This again displays an awareness of the patient's position.

On line 16, the patient displays that, as yet, he is not quite comfortable with taking the proactive role and choosing a name. After the 0.4 second pause on line 15, rather than volunteering a name that he would like to use, the patient asks: 'W'll what do you prefer'. In order to maintain a non-directive stance here the practitioner has to continue to leave the choosing of the name up to the patient. So, on line 17, the practitioner hedges, saying 'Ye- (.) wh- you just wh- any way you want'. By not making a choice for the patient, the doctor also sets another precedent. In a subtle pre-echo of the self-empowerment that is so important in holistic medicine, his reticence conveys the message that the patient is able (required almost) to take an active role in deciding what is right for him – even at this basic level. It also helps to establish the authenticity of possible future choices that may arise by serving as a concrete demonstration of respect for the patient's preferences.

By line 19, the patient is still unwilling to commit to a name and produces a short burst of laughter with which the practitioner overlaps 'Okay . . . what do you like to be called wh-' (lines 20–1). This is, again, a significant move: in choosing to turn the question around, the doctor not only avoids making the choice himself, but also manages to convert the sequence into something empowering for the patient. By asking the patient a question that he will almost certainly answer, and which allows him to demonstrate a definite and self-supplied preference, the disjunctive flavour of the previous sequence is largely counteracted. Most significant here, however, is the way in which the doctor's request is framed to elicit the patient's first name. When asked 'what do you like to be called', the patient is unlikely to produce a formal title such as 'Mr Smith', the default will be 'Billy'. This has the effect of subtly establishing that first names can be used from then on.

This naming sequence demonstrates how the creative use of alternative or tangential moves by the health professional can rescue sequences that have become 'stuck', without the need for an abandonment of the topic. Peräkylä (1995) for example, outlines how, in family systems therapy (which routinely involves two co-counsellors), this may be achieved by the intervention of the second counsellor. The similarity here is that these interventions frequently seem to involve the asking of a question that offers a way out for the client but that preserves the activity in hand (Peräkylä 1995). In this case, as well as preserving the activity of deciding on names, the practitioner's turn in lines 20–1 also has the effect of defusing a situation in which the patient might begin to come across as unco-operative; he is not placed in a position where he appears to be continually blocking, or not aligning with, the practitioner. By avoiding the perpetuation of a disjunctive sequence the practitioner continues to build the feeling that he respects the patient's wishes and preferences. In a broader sense too, the naming sequence begins to project a kind of extended temporality; it helps to frame the current encounter in the context of a longer ongoing process in which names, and the levels of intimacy associated with the various levels of formality that they imply, will be important.

In conventional consultations, although doctors obviously routinely introduce themselves to patients, it might be unusual to find this much attention being given to naming options:

> **Extract 9**
> I mean, [it's] not based on any science but of an age or just appearance or my own personal prejudice as well, which one [I use]. One is slightly more informal than the other. What is interesting is what people choose to call me. I don't lay down any rule, I'll respond to anything. It is interesting what people, particularly sort of repeat patients will end up calling, some refer to you still as doctor or Dr Smith and some people will call me by my first name, and I don't know how they decide that or why they decide that, it's a mystery to me. I still like to keep it slightly more formal, that's why when I introduce myself it's either John Smith or Doctor. But the way that you name yourself can have a bearing on the rapport and the formality. Other than that it's straight down, you know, the first question then is, 'Well, what can we do for you?' – straight into that.
>
> (GP, themed discussion)

Although this doctor is concerned that the way in which 'naming' is enacted will have an effect on the rapport he is able to generate with his patients, this is not foremost in his mind. His main focus is on ascertaining the patient's presenting complaint. In terms of empirical data, a similarly 'standard' approach to naming in an orthodox consultation is given in Extract 10, taken from the opening of a consultation in a cancer genetics clinic:

Extract 10 (D = doctor; P = patient)

```
D:  Well Mrs Jones, as I said welcome to the genetics
    clinic, ·hh and I'm Doctor Brown, and ahm (0.3) . .
    this is a clinic where we see folks with (0.5)
    something in the family.
P:  Yes
D:  Sometimes people are born with a problem ·hh and
    folks are wondering what is- tha:t it can happen
    again.
```

(Consultation in clinical genetics, Y-202-207)

This sequence is taken from the beginning of a consultation with a new patient at a genetics outpatient clinic. Rather than an extended two-way interaction, the doctor simply greets the patient and gives her own name. There is an assumed level of formality in the use of the patient's married name by the doctor, and similarly, the practitioner refers to herself as 'Doctor Brown'. Other naming options are not offered, and within the same turn as this introduction the doctor begins to focus on a description of what goes on at the clinic: '. . . I'm Doctor Brown . . . this is a clinic where we see folks with (0.5) something in the family' (lines 2–3). This is not to suggest that this approach is somehow inferior or wrong, rather, it illustrates how variations in opportunities for patients to become involved begin with the most basic aspects of interaction. It seems that the practitioner in our case study is more sensitive to how the conventions associated with naming in the medical encounter might perpetuate structural inequalities – inequalities which in conventional medical encounters such as the one quoted in Extract 10 might not be considered particularly significant – but which could be a barrier to the generation of a rapport, and which could, by implication, affect the quality of the information that the patient gives. By conveying that, although this is a medical encounter, the issue of how the parties might address each other does not have to follow conventional rules, the practitioner in Extract 8 is in effect asking the patient to begin looking at the consultation process in a different way. If the patient is aware that, even in the most basic way, markers in his internalized model of a medical consultation are subject to alteration, he can start to abandon, or at least to question, what the encounter should look like. He may then become more receptive to the balanced interaction that the holistic process seeks to engender.

Developing rapport

At the end of the naming sequence (line 25) there is some overt evidence of a rapport developing between the doctor and the patient. The generation of rapport and empathy is regarded as being extremely important to the success of the therapeutic process in all consultations (Mercer et al. 2004); and is often emphasized by homoeopaths:

> **Extract 11**
>
> [I]t's crucial with homoeopathy because you're building a relationship with the patient. It all hinges on that really, being able to understand the patient, them feeling relaxed with you, being able to fully convey what is happening for them. Being able to empathize with someone I'm sure helps [the patient] to feel understood. Empathy and rapport are very important in homoeopathy – rapport in the sense that you are able to understand somebody, but empathy is the depth with which you can understand them. Rapport could be

more of a – almost like a conversational style, that you're speaking the same language – but empathy is on a much deeper emotional level.

(Homoeopath, themed discussion)

Although obviously important in the context of conventional medical consultations in the sense that they represent 'successful' communication between a doctor and a patient, in orthodox settings such as primary care, empathy and rapport can be seen as having less of a functional role (and see Peräkylä et al., Chapter 7, this volume). That is, they can be regarded as helpful interactional states (Coulehan et al. 2001), but without the same 'diagnostic' importance as in homoeopathy:

Extract 12

[Y]es, they're important, it would be difficult to say they're not important. Certainly, rapport would seem to be important to my mind. The basic tool that you have is, apart from the medication, is the consultation so that's important, and if you don't have rapport and by that I mean, an easy way of discussing things with people and they with you, then that consultation is going to be very difficult and you're not going to get all the information that you need. So I would place rapport as extremely important. Empathy? Empathy, I struggle with a little bit but I guess unless you have empathy it might be difficult to have rapport and so far as people pick up on [if] you're being superficial and not particularly interested – interest being one component of empathy, if you like – if you're not interested, people pick up on that.

(GP, themed discussion)

Significantly, in Extract 8, the fragment of talk that evokes the sense of developing rapport is initiated by the patient rather than the practitioner. The patient makes a humorous comment relating to the prior talk about his name: '°Er:° (0.4) my wife's got various names for me °(though)° . . .' Apart from the therapeutically grounded reasons for the successful generation of rapport highlighted by the homeopath in Extract 6, it can also be important in terms of displaying overt equality within the interaction; turns at talk or behavioural routines that directly indicate a rapport need not be limited to the practitioner, but can equally be initiated by the patient.

The times at which rapport or empathy are evident in actual talk routines, in any medical setting, can be seen as high points when the socio-emotional undercurrent breaks the surface of the surrounding interaction and becomes focused on a particular sequence of behaviour. Even if a consultation generates the overall impression of mutuality, and the parties are aware of a rapport, there may only be a couple of 'peaks' during the ongoing talk when these states are definitely in play. The picture may be further complicated by rapport and empathy being occasionally marked by an *absence* of talk or overt interaction. Kacperek (1997), for example, in reflecting on how her nursing practice was affected by losing her voice, related that this apparent disability actually enhanced her ability to generate empathetic relationships with patients. Presumably, however, the cumulative effect of mutualistic spoken behaviours that are consistently in tune with the generation of these states (such as the reference to the camera and naming sequences), keep them near the surface where they can reflexively permeate the ongoing interaction.

Certain kinds of behaviour, such as the patient's attempt at a humorous aside (line 25), not only serve to indicate that a rapport may be developing, but can also be regarded as prompts by one party for a verification of the new interactional dynamic. Even though it may be the practitioner who has steered the interaction to a position where there is a certain amount of sub-textual connection, either party may initiate the verification. It may, as in this case, be the patient who actually risks a turn that brings it into the open. The 'risk', for whoever tries to concretize the rapport, is that they may have misjudged the degree to which the other party is projecting receptiveness; remember that at this stage in the interaction, neither party has had more than a couple of minutes to evaluate each other. In initiating a turn that in effect asks for confirmation that they may now move to another level of intimacy, the person who does this leaves themselves open to rejection – in this case, the patient risks their joke falling flat. This is reflected in the way he delivers his turn. Line 25 has a flavour of experimentation, of testing the water; the initial '°Er:°' is spoken quietly and followed by a relatively long interval of 0.4 seconds. Similarly, the final part of the comment: '. . . me °(though)°' is attenuated. These dynamics help to emphasize a feeling that the patient is not entirely sure about the appropriateness of his comment, or the response he will receive. There is a rhetorical quality to the line too, which, had the practitioner failed to give a reciprocal response, would have allowed the patient a degree of face-saving. A comment like this, spoken almost as an aside to oneself, does not depend on a response from the other party. In fact, here, the patient's comment generates laughter from the practitioner: '^KH ·<ha-ha>' (line 27). This is significant, because the doctor then proceeds, from his laughter, to build on the patient's 'joke'. After an aside ('. . . °picked up a pen that doesn't work – there it is° . . .') the doctor produces a collusive follow-up, saying: '°I bet you she does°' (line 28). The way in which this part of the turn is spoken, with a quiet, almost conspiratorial tone, deepens the sense of fellowship between the two parties and hints at the beginnings of a deeper rapport. His '°I bet you she does°' seems to briefly shift the interaction into a different mode, one that is almost intimate. Like the patient's feed line, this too has a 'testing' quality, as if the practitioner allows his professional persona to drop for a second, but quickly restores it. He lets the patient see that more intimate dynamics are acceptable, without overtly pushing the interaction in that direction. The comment has an authentic 'I know what you mean' quality, but is subtle enough not to rush the acclimatization of the patient. The short laugh that follows the comment ('^k-h ·-hu', line 29) has a similarly attenuated quality, but is again perfectly matched to the feel of the sequence; too hearty a laugh here may have come across as false, whereas no laugh at all might have given the practitioner's comment a slightly sarcastic edge.

Deeper socialization

The final activity we would like to examine pushes the expectations of behaviour in this consultation setting a little further. It is not uncommon for a health care professional to go through a process of explaining to a new patient 'ground rules' such as confidentiality, trust, openness, and so on, although the cultural assumptions that come with visiting a GP or a surgeon in a clinic might make this kind of activity relatively rare. In medical encounters to which the patient is accustomed and which have become relatively routine, these elements can be taken largely for granted. If they need to be highlighted for any reason, simply talking about them might be a perfectly sufficient means of communicating them. In a homoeopathic hospital setting that is new to the patient, however, there may be little in the way of background cultural knowledge for the patient to fall back on, so along with words, the practical behaviour of the practitioner can help to convey elements of holism. By ensuring that, early on, the patient is exposed to examples of the practitioner *actually performing* behavioural routines that demonstrate trust, openness, respect, and so on, and that directly involve the patient, the essence of the holistic approach can be quickly communicated in a tangible way.

Immediately following the naming sequence in Extract 8, the practitioner engages in an activity that is an extremely good example of this. On line 29, after the 0.7 second pause, he indicates that he would like to re-read the referral letter sent by the patient's GP. The patient, naturally enough, concurs with this and for the next 20 seconds or so the practitioner carefully studies the letter. What is interesting is that once he has done this, he says: 'tk- ·h actually maybe I could read you the letter out' (line 35). Also, the way in which the doctor qualifies his action is significant. On line 39, he says: 'That will let you know what I know', in a concrete example of his use of the principles of transparency and mutualism that he is trying to convey to the patient. Similarly, as the patient is acknowledging that this is acceptable ('Right', line 40), the practitioner continues '. . . then we can kick off on the story' (lines 39 and 41). This, again, reinforces affiliation and equality because it casts the information in the letter (and by implication, the patient's other/past medical experiences) as less relevant than the interactions that the practitioner and patient will subsequently share. It communicates that in this new environment it is the patient's story that is important, not what his doctors may have said about him in the past. The use of the word *story* helps to begin subtly socializing the patient into regarding the encounter as an arena in which narrative and subjectivity are welcome.

The implied equalizing of the practitioner–patient dynamic that starts on line 39 is further echoed once the doctor has completed his narration of the referral letter. On lines 65–7 he says: 'So that's what I . . . know so far ·hh so you kick off at any point you want really with the story'. Again his repeated use of the word *story* builds on the feeling of holism – he does not ask specifically focused symptomatic questions but rather prompts the patient to think of his problem as part of a wider life narrative. There is a sense too that the practitioner is casting himself and the patient as co-workers who have equal rights in deciding the direction of the interaction. The practitioner's directive role, in his professional capacity, is significantly downplayed; he actively hands the decision (about where to begin the story) over to the patient and provides no prompts to indicate which elements might be of significance. By sharing information that might normally be unavailable to the patient, the practitioner is demonstrating in a practical way that his approach embodies openness and transparency. In the same way that, once he offered a name choice to the patient he left the decision open and avoided making it for him, reading out the letter and the reasons he gives for doing this become tangible proof of his integrity. His words are backed by action – he literally does let the patient know what he knows. This particular practitioner may be in some respects extreme in his approach to openness. On other occasions when we observed his consultations, he would show patients pages from their notes if he felt this would help make something clearer for them (see also Ruusuvuori 2005; Peräkylä et al., Chapter 7, this volume).

Conclusion

In this chapter we have tried to give a flavour of some elements that contribute to the creation of a mutualistic and interactionally balanced atmosphere in a consultation, with reference to the opening sequences of one video-recorded case. Our analyses are necessarily exploratory: they are based on a single case, and are concerned with the identification and description of particular elements of the interaction that appear to engender a feeling of equality. In illustrating these elements, we have sought to show how they can promote the patient's participation; how they can create the conditions for participation, and thus perhaps enable patients to talk about their concerns and needs. We have focused on the initial transition period into the start of the consultation proper, highlighting environmental and interactional features that have relevance for patient's feelings of comfort and ease in any health care situation they find themselves in. We have sought to show that studying the interactional mechanisms of a holistic approach to health care that combines orthodox and complementary systems may therefore be a useful means by which those often hidden structural and procedural elements of medical encounters, which influence the enactment of patient-centredness, can be exposed. These often hidden elements, when made more overt, may offer ways of increasing patients' opportunities for participation, as well as supplying examples for health care professionals in training as to how to promote participation.

This chapter has focused on elements that will resonate with conventional and complementary medicine practitioners – consultation environment, mutuality, rapport, and so on. By studying the merging of homoeopathic and conventional medical practice in one consultation, analysis of interaction at a micro-level within the consultation setting can be particularly useful. It is one area where there can be a degree of crossover and constructive dialogue between systems that are routinely polarized. Most significantly, perhaps, it provides a means through which health professionals' communication practices, in the most routine and commonplace of consultation activities, can be made explicit, and may therefore be taught (and see the Educational Supplement, pp. 205–7, for some examples).

Acknowledgement

Some of the data in this chapter were originally collected for a research project on patient participation in decision-making (reference 3700514), funded by the Department of Health: Health in Partnership Programme (see Farrell 2004). The analysis presented here is the original work of the authors and the opinions may not be shared by that research project or by the funding body.

Recommendations: summary

- By studying apparently commonplace routines such as introductions, qualities that help to build rapport and to establish a relationship between the patient and the health professional are uncovered.
- Close description of a single case from one consultation embodying a holistic, integrated medicine approach reveals a repertoire of communication behaviours that invite the patient's active participation.
- By focusing on the details of interaction in particular types of consultations, it is possible to locate points of similarity and contrast between health care approaches that can generate dialogue and exchange of ideas between them concerning patients' participation.

6 Patient participation in formulating and opening sequences

Joseph Gafaranga and Nicky Britten

Commentary

This chapter continues the strand of investigation begun in Chapter 5 into the details of interaction between patients and health professionals and how these facilitate the process of participation. Based on a data set of general practice consultations recorded in the UK, it considers two consultation activities: initial concern elicitors in opening sequences, and formulations of patients' problems. The former invites comparison with the opening of a therapeutic holistic medicine encounter (see Chapter 5); the latter invites comparison with the responses that patients produce to psychoanalysts' interpretations (see Chapter 7) which may be considered as one type of formulation.

In order to explore questions concerning patient participation and how particular activities shape the forms patient participation can take, this chapter adopts a critical perspective on the relation between linguistic form and pragmatic functions, and on theories of professional interaction. From this starting point, this chapter demonstrates three specific contributions that detailed description of interaction, as it unfolds sequentially, can make to the study of patient participation. One, it enables a view of participation which, rather than consisting of linguistic forms, begins with activities and pragmatic functions. Two, it adopts a participants' perspective in determining which activities are significant and which are not. Three, it allows patients' and health professionals' actions in consultations to be considered in their sequential environment.

The analyses of instances of the two activities (the opening sequence and formulations of the patient's problem) show a number of ways in which patients influence the definition and discussion of their presenting problem.

Generalizing from these instances, the issue of whether 'improved' participation can be obtained within the current consultation format, or whether a new structure of the consultation as a cultural event needs to be made available, is discussed. Finally, this chapter argues that in order to measure patient participation and to recommend training for health professionals in it, it is important to be clear about the particular ways of talking and forms of participation with which our research is concerned.

Introduction

As described elsewhere in this book, the UK Government is promoting citizen involvement through its modernization agenda of inclusiveness, stakeholder engagement and partnership working (see Chapter 3). Community-level initiatives such as Patient and Public Involvement have been undertaken, but there is also a strong expectation that involvement must be observed at the level of the consultation (see Chapter 1). Thus, the term patient involvement, or participation, is now common. However, the concept of patient participation itself, especially when it is used to refer to the patient's involvement in the consultation, is little understood. Rather, it is often taken for granted, as self-explanatory. To clarify this situation, Peräkylä and Vehviläinen's (2003) notion of 'professional stocks of interactional knowledge' (SIK) is a useful one. According to Peräkylä and Vehviläinen (2003: 729), these stocks of interactional knowledge are 'models and theories or quasi-theories about interaction' held by practitioners as 'part of their knowledge base'. We suggest that patient participation could be a part of one such SIK.

Peräkylä and Vehviläinen (2003) and Peräkylä et al. (2005) divide research into doctor–patient interaction into three categories. As regards patient participation, this distinction is very relevant. On the one hand, there are studies (for example, Roter 1977; Cegala et al. 2000; Street and Millay 2001) which are 'produced from within the profession (and therefore for which) the SIK provides central theoretical concepts in terms of which empirical data are articulated' (Peräkylä and Vehviläinen 2003: 730). In these studies, the concept of patient participation is taken to be self-evident; all that needs to be done is to measure it quantitatively. On the other hand, there are conversation analysis (CA) studies of doctor–patient interaction which 'focus on the structures and practices of interaction per se' (Peräkylä and Vehviläinen 2003: 730) and which are not concerned with issues of patient participation as such. In between these two, there is a third perspective, also CA-based: one which 'focuses on sequential structures of interaction and seeks a dialogue with the SIKs' (Peräkylä and Vehviläinen 2003: 730; see for example, Stivers and Heritage 2001; Stivers 2002; Robinson 2003). Typically, studies in this third category describe a particular structure or practice of social interaction in detail and consider the implications for patient participation.

In this chapter, we will adopt this third perspective. That is, we look at two interactional practices we have described elsewhere and, in each case, ask two specific questions:

1 What does patient participation mean?
2 How can patient participation be improved?

The specific interactional practices we look at are: formulation in general practice consultations (Gafaranga and Britten 2004), and the opening sequence in general practice consultations (Gafaranga and Britten 2003; 2005). The rationale for this methodological choice is that, as detailed by Peräkylä and Vehviläinen (2003: 731–2), CA can relate to SIKs in four different ways:

1 CA *falsifies and corrects* assumptions that are part of a SIK.
2 CA *provides a more detailed picture* of practices that are described in a SIK.
3 CA *adds a new dimension* to the understanding of practices described by a SIK.
4 CA *expands the description* of practices provided by a SIK and suggests some missing links between the SIK and the interactional practices (original emphasis).

Our aim in this chapter is to show how, by focusing on specific interactional activities, we can begin to develop a detailed understanding of the concept of patient participation.

Patient participation and professional stocks of interactional knowledge

As we have indicated above, most current accounts of communication in the consultation, apart from those carried out by conversation analysts, do not aim to understand the concept of patient participation *per se*. This is partly because, as others have pointed out (see Cegala et al. 2000; Drew 2001), relatively little attention has been given to *patients'* contributions to medical discourse. Instead, research has tended to focus on physicians' behaviour (and see Chapter 1, this volume). Thus, the meta-analysis of provider behaviour carried out by Hall et al. (1988) identified five broad categories of physician communication: (information giving, question asking, partnership building, rapport building and socio-emotional talk). Stewart et al.'s (1995) influential model of patient-centred medicine highlights six 'interactive components', all of which refer to the professional's tasks and behaviours. Elwyn et al.'s (2003b) instrument for measuring shared decision-making, the OPTION scale, has 12 items relating to the clinician's behaviour. When the patient's contribution is considered, it tends to be categorized into parallel categories to the physician's contribution. Thus, Roter and Hall (1992) identified specific variables in patients' patterns of talk: information giving, information receiving, social conversation, positive talk and negative talk. The use of these fixed categories facilitates quantitative research and statistical analysis of relationships between variables; it also facilitates the teaching and learning of communication skills by identifying discrete tasks for the student to master.

Notwithstanding this focus on health professional behaviour, notions of patient participation are often present in the literature, if only implicitly. Thus, in contrasting the biomedical and disease context with the integrated illness context that incorporates the patient perspective, Roter (2000) is implying that patient participation can influence the content of the consultation. In defining the participatory nature of relationship-centred care, she claims that physicians have a responsibility and obligation to help patients assume an 'authentic and responsible role' in the medical dialogue. She goes on to say that a teacher helps by equipping learners (patients) with what they need to help themselves. Cegala et al. (2000) carried out one of the few intervention studies explicitly aimed at increasing patients' participation in medical interviews, through processes of information exchange. They measured patient participation using ten variables categorized under three headings: information seeking, information provision, and information verifying. Some of these variables included an interactive element, for example, 'solicited replies' in the category of information provision. However, generally speaking, these variables did not code the interactions between patients and physicians. In general, the use of pre-assigned categories such as these can be problematic. Little account is taken of the interactive elements, in other words, the ways in which one person's talk is occasioned by, or oriented to, what the other person has said (or not said). No account is taken either of the immediate context of the talk or of what the speaker is achieving through their talk.

One of the few papers to give an explicit definition of patient participation is that of Street and Millay (2001), whose definition we use as a point of comparison for our own work. They write:

> for our purpose, we define patient participation as the extent to which patients produce verbal responses that have the potential to significantly influence the content and structure of the interaction as well as the health care provider's beliefs and behaviours.
>
> (2001: 62)

Central to their approach is the notion of 'verbal acts of participation'.

According to Street and Millay (2001: 62–3), these verbal acts of participation include 'asking questions, descriptions of health experiences, expressions of concern, giving opinions, making suggestions, stating preferences'. More precisely, three types of acts are identified as 'essential and observable features of patient participation in medical encounters'; namely, asking questions, expressing concerns and assertive utterances. Summary definitions of each of these categories are presented in Table 6.1 (from Street and Millay 2001: 63).

There are various respects in which these definitions can be commented on, but, here, we will just mention three problems they present, for understanding patient participation. The first problem has to do with the very definition of patient participation. According to Street and Millay, there is participation if the patient's action has 'the potential to significantly influence the content and structure of the interaction as well as the health care provider's beliefs and behaviours'. Clearly, this definition is not particularly useful, since, as CA studies have shown, any action by one participant, including silence, has the potential to affect subsequent actions by co-participants (and see Chapter 7). This is the very basis of the notion of 'sequentiality' (Drew et al. 2001; Wooffitt 2001). In other words, the definition can be paraphrased as: every verbal action by the patient is an act of participation. And, if this is the case, it is not clear what the definition is meant to achieve.

Table 6.1 Street and Millay's (2001) operational definition of communicative acts of patient participation

Verbal behaviour	*Definition*	*Examples*
Asking questions	Utterances in interrogative form intended to seek information and clarification	'What's my thyroid?' 'Does smoking cause that?' 'Is there anything they can do?'
Expressions of concern	Utterances in which the patient expresses worry, anxiety, fear, anger, frustration, and other forms of negative affect or emotions	'It's very frustrating' 'No, . . . I just have a fear of the operation' 'I'm even scared to play with my own grand-daughter'
Assertive responses	Utterances in which the patient expresses his or her rights, beliefs, interests, and desires as in offering an opinion, stating preferences, making suggestions or recommendations, disagreeing, or interrupting	'Go ahead and do it' 'I really don't want anybody to x-ray it' 'I don't want to have to lie for it'

The second problem with the above definitions relates to the inconsistencies they show and the relationship they imply between linguistic form and pragmatic function. For example, the category 'asking questions' is defined with reference to the linguistic form of the utterances used, while neither of the other two types of acts is defined in this way. According to Street and Millay, to count as the act of 'asking a question', an utterance has to be in the interrogative form. Reading through the examples given for the other two categories, one gets a definite impression that, to count either as an expression of concern or as an assertive response, an utterance must be in the declarative form. However, Speech Acts Theory (Austin 1962; Searle 1969) has shown that there is no direct link between linguistic forms and pragmatic functions. For example, to seek information or clarification, one need not use an interrogative form (Cegala et al. 2000). Likewise, a worry can be expressed as a question, just as an expression of preference (assertive response) can take the form of a question. Consider Extract 1, from Britten et al. (2004). In their paper, Britten et al. demonstrate that, in its actual context, the highlighted element (lines 5–6) is an expression of preference (aversion to medicine). However, as the transcript shows, this utterance has, grammatically, taken the interrogative form. Note that a potential 'misunderstanding' has occurred here, in that the doctor interprets the patient's utterance literally, as a question, and responds to it as such (line 7):

Extract 1 (D = doctor; P = patient)

```
D:  [Oh right
P:  [And when I told her I'd got it again she says You ain't
    been taking your tablets =
D:  [Yeah
P:  [cos Dad keeps having to take- Have I got to
    [keep taking them?
D:  [That's right. You've got to keep taking at least one a day.
    (0.1) Okay
```

(Audio-recorded consultation in general practice, GP3P10)

In her question in lines 5–6, the patient implies that taking the tablets may be uncomfortable for her, and in this sense she also expresses an aversion to the medication being talked about. Thus, the patient's turn at talk is not only a question but also an expression of preference. That is to say, in order to understand patient participation, one must start, not from linguistic forms, but rather from functions which are actually expressed and actions which are actually accomplished.

The third problem, following from the above, is that Street and Millay's pragmatic approach can easily fail to capture significant acts of patient participation, as in Extract 2:

Extract 2

```
1  D:  right. okay. And what can I do for you today?
2  P:  you - my blood test er from er my gout ((laughs))
3  D:  right. yes. yes. Yes. Th:e uric acid is- is high
4  P:  is it. Yeah
```

(Audio-recorded consultation in general practice, GP3P11)

In Street and Millay, it is not clear how the highlighted turn will be analysed. It is not a question, and nor is it an expression of concern of the kind illustrated in Street and Millay and, although it is a response to the doctor's question in turn 1, it can hardly be seen as an assertive one. It is not an expression of 'rights, beliefs, interests, desires, etc.'. On the other hand, when the talk is observed closely, it is clear that the patient's utterance in line 2 is a highly significant act of participation and that it has been interpreted as such by the doctor himself. In line 3, the doctor responds to the patient's talk as having served to remind him ('right . . . yes yes') of something ('the uric acid is high'); see below for an analysis of this example. In other words, to understand the patient's participation, one must look at the patient's contributions in line 2 in its sequential environment.

Briefly, these limitations of the pragmatic approach point to the need to do the following:

- view patient participation as consisting, not of linguistic forms, but of activities and pragmatic functions;
- adopt a participant's perspective in determining which actions are significant and which are not;
- consider acts in their sequential environment.

An interactional activities perspective on patient participation

As stated in the introduction to this chapter, in addition to SIK-based research, patient participation has also been examined by CA studies of doctor–patient interaction. Some contributions of CA, as an approach to talk as social action, are discussed and referenced in Chapter 1. As we have already indicated in this chapter, with respect to patient participation, CA-based studies divide into two categories. The category of interest here is those studies that describe interactional structures and draw implications for patient participation. Two types of implications are drawn. Some studies highlight structural constraints on patient participation. For example, Robinson (2003) demonstrates ways in which patient participation is constrained by the overall structure of interaction during GP consultations for acute problems. Other studies show that consultation and conversational structures offer opportunities for patient participation (as detailed in Chapter 1). To mention just one here, Stivers (2005a) shows how, because treatment recommendations normatively require patients' agreement, they provide a structural opportunity for patient participation.

In line with this tradition of research, our aim in this chapter is to show that, by focusing on specific interactional activities, we might begin to develop a detailed understanding of the concept of patient participation. The first interactional activity we will look at is 'formulation'. Broadly speaking, formulation can be described as the activity of restating/rephrasing something that has already been said in the conversation.

Formulation and patient participation

In their Information Exchange model of patient participation, Cegala et al. (2000) recognize formulation as one specific verbal act of patient participation and more precisely as an 'information-verifying' act. From a CA perspective, 'formulations are a means through which participants may make explicit their sense of "what we are talking about" or "what was just said": they are a means for constructing an explicit sense of the gist of the talk thus far' (Drew 2003: 296). In a study based on GP consultations (Gafaranga and Britten 2004), we analysed formulations with regard to their focus, location and function in the consultation, and made three observations concerning the properties of formulations that may be significant for an understanding of patient participation. The first of these observations is that a distinction must be made between self-formulation and other-formulation. In self-formulation, a participant (doctor or patient) formulates their own talk; in other-formulation, they formulate the co-participant's talk. Both types of formulation can be found in Extract 3. In line 6, the doctor formulates the 'gist' (Heritage and Watson 1979) of the patient's talk and, in line 7, the patient formulates his own talk:

Extract 3

1 D: Okay. <Curtains drawn back> Well if you're drinking
2 eight pints of beer every day-
3 P: Well not every day (is it). On average.
4 D: On average
5 P: Average yeah
6 D: **So sometimes you drink more and sometimes you drink less**
7 P: **And sometimes I don't drink at all** ((talk continues))

(Audio-recorded consultation in general practice, GP16P43)

The second observation regarding the properties of formulation concerns the need to distinguish between what we have called 'formulating summaries' and 'action formulation'. A formulating summary summarizes 'the talk on topic-in-progress', that is, it looks back at the talk immediately preceding it. Both formulations in Extract 3 are instances of formulating summaries, because they express the participants' understanding of the directly preceding talk, on the topic of the patient's alcohol use. An action formulation, on the other hand, looks back at the action previously agreed upon in the consultation, and may be 'distant from the section of talk it formulates' (Gafaranga and Britten 2004: 155). Consider Extract 4. The formulation in line 3 restates an action which has been agreed upon almost a hundred turns earlier in the consultation:

Extract 4

1 D: ((uses computer)) And some Lactulose
2 P: Yes.
3 D: Right. And **so just swap the Zantac for this new one**
4 P: Yes
5 D: And see how you get on

(Audio-recorded consultation in general practice, GP4P11)

Our third observation concerns the functionality dimension of formulation and its significance for understanding patient participation. In doctor–patient interaction, formulation has both a cognitive and an organizational function. Cognitive function refers to the role that formulation plays in the negotiation of understanding between participants; and organizational function to the role of formulation in the sequencing of activities in interaction. At the cognitive level, other-formulating summaries reveal the speaker's understanding of co-participant's talk (see line 6, Extract 3); while, through self-formulating summaries, speakers reveal how their own talk is to be understood (see line 7, Extract 3). Extract 3 is particularly interesting in this respect, as the participants do not share the same understanding. As can be gathered from lines 1–2, the doctor has formed the impression that the patient's problems are a result of his heavy drinking while the patient contests this interpretation (line 3). These diverging positions are further played out in the formulating sequence. The patient acts as if completing the list (Jefferson 1990) that the doctor has started ('So sometimes you drink more and sometimes you drink less') while with his completion ('And sometimes I don't drink at all'), he undermines the doctor's interpretation. The function of information verifying (Cegala et al. 2000) actually derives from this possibility of other-formulating summary. Through formulation, participants display their understanding of ongoing talk and open that understanding up for evaluation by co-participants. In turn, in view of the displayed understanding, the co-participant takes the appropriate next action and either agrees or disagrees with the displayed understanding.

An action formulation by the doctor can be used to confirm that a patient commits (renews their commitment) to a course of action already agreed in the consultation. Conversely, action formulation by the patient can be used as a strategy whereby, *of their own initiative*, the patient confirms their agreement and commitment to the proposed course of action (Gafaranga and Britten 2004: 166). An instance of action formulation by the doctor is provided in Extract 4, where the doctor returns to the treatment recommendation that has already been agreed upon. An instance of action formulation by the patient is provided in Extract 5. As the transcript shows, in line 7, the patient formulates the treatment recommendation which has been agreed upon earlier in the interaction:

Extract 5

1 P: Right. So what do I do about this then?
2 D: Take that to front desk
3 P: Oh do I. Right.
4 D: and er the [girls'll make an appointment for you=
5 P: [Okay
6 = [to see her
7 P: [Lovely. Jolly good. **So just lavender oil and ice.**
8 D: Yes
9 P: Right. Thanks very much
10 D: That's all right
11 P: Best of luck [for the rest of the day
12 D: [Ta ta
13 P: Bye

(Audio-recorded consultation in general practice, GP11P37)

Thus, Extracts 4 and 5 show how either participant may use formulations to ensure that they have reached a shared understanding on the course of action to be taken after the consultation.

In addition to their cognitive function, formulations serve an organizational function. In doctor–patient interaction, formulation is closing-implicative. Formulating summaries announce imminent exit from a topic-in-progress (Button 1991) while action formulation announces exit from the consultation as a whole. Consider Extract 6:

Extract 6 (D = doctor; M = mother; P = patient)

1 D: when did they actually sta:rt?
2 M: Er- [it was February
3 D: [Do you actually remember?
4 P: It was February
5 D: [so two-

P: [Not this February the February before
M: Two years this February
D: **So it's been two years**
P: Yeah
D: yeah
M: Mm
D: Yeah. Th- as I say these- these first couple of years
erm the- the- beginning and ending the periods
M: Mm
D: Things often a- a few- few years sometimes to get into a
pattern

(Audio-recorded consultation in general practice, GP10P32)

In this consultation, a young woman is consulting about a number of problems, including painful periods. Her mother is also present. The main task at hand in the sequence above is to establish how long the patient has been having periods. In line 1, the doctor initiates the sequence with a question. Over the next few turns (lines 2–7), the participants work out the answer to the question. In line 8, the doctor uses a formulation to reveal his understanding of the worked-out answer. Then, in a series of turns (lines 9–11), the participants each display their agreement as to the adequacy of the answer to the question presented by the doctor in line 1 and, by implication, their orientation to the completeness of the sequence. This orientation is shared by the doctor, who initiates another sub-topic in line 12. Likewise, in Extract 5, in line 7, the patient looks back at the consultation and, as if to say 'this is what I take away with me', formulates the agreed course of action and, after confirmation by the doctor, launches the closing episode.

Briefly, formulation is more than just an 'information-verifying' strategy. By implication, at this level, patient participation is more than using formulation to verify information. Rather, participation by means of formulation consists of using it effectively in all its different aspects. This includes patients producing self-formulating summaries in order to show the main point of their own talk, recognizing other-formulating summaries as displays of understanding, and reacting appropriately. Participation at this level also means patients recognizing the professional's organizational agenda when they produce formulations. Failing to do so may lead to frustrations and a feeling of being interrupted. Patient participation at the level of action formulation means that the patient recognizes the function of formulation when used by the doctor. When used by the doctor, action formulation is essentially an undertaking to 'reinforce an already achieved agreement between the parties, to get the patient to renew his or her commitment to doing what has been agreed' (Gafaranga and Britten 2004: 165). This is significant because, as our data have shown, doctors can use the strategy even when there has not been any agreement. Patient participation in such cases therefore means to recognize and resist this 'manipulation' if this becomes necessary. But patient participation also means for the patient to be able to tell the doctor that they agree to the treatment plan they have negotiated together. Action formulation is an efficient way of doing this.

Patient participation and the opening sequence

Our second interactional activity is the opening of a consultation as described in Gafaranga and Britten (2003; 2005). Looking at general practice consultations, we observed that, overwhelmingly, they open with what we referred to as a 'first concern elicitor'. We also observed that a variety of concern elicitors (see Gafaranga and Britten 2005: 79) are available for doctors to use, including 'How are you?', 'What can I do for you?', 'How are you getting on?', and 'What brings you here today?'. Given this diversity, we wanted to know if the choice of elicitors was random or whether there was some order to it.

Observation of the data revealed that doctors and patients had a 'scheme of interpretation' (Garfinkel 1967) guiding their acts. They defined each consultation either as a new consultation or as a follow-up consultation. A new consultation was one in which patients presented with a new problem and a follow-up consultation was one in which they presented with a problem the doctor was (assumed to be) already aware of. When the doctor presented the consultation as a follow-up, they used 'How are you?' and its variants to invite the patient to display their reason for the visit. Extract 7 illustrates this possibility. Evidence that, in this consultation, both participants agree on its definition as a follow-up can be found in 'retrospective tying devices' (Firth 1995: 188) such as the modifiers 'my/your' and the comparative form 'better'. By saying 'my cold' and not, say, 'I have a cold', it is as if the patient is saying 'the cold you know of'. Likewise, by saying 'better', the patient seems to be saying 'compared to what it was last time':

Extract 7

1 D: That's fine. Well **how are you?**
2 P: **My** cold's much **better**
3 D: Your cold's [much better
4 P: [much better

(Audio-recorded consultation in general practice, GP4P8)

Conversely, when the consultation was defined as new, 'What can I do for you?' and its variants were used. Extract 8 is an example:

Extract 8

D: sorry to keep you. had an [interesting afternoon?
P: [oh that's all right
D: have a chair (0.3) now that thyroid test I did in March
April was normal wasn't it
P: [yeah
D: **[what can I do for you today?**
P: Er (.) couple of things. (0.2) Night before last (0.3) I
was inveigled into our field to pull thistles out.
D: [oh
P: [cos it was so wet it'd be a doddle to pull them out
D: mm
P: an it was. So there I was bending down among grass which
was erm in flower
D: mm
P: and I woke up in the night with erm really uncomfortable
hay fever=
D: mm
P: =symptoms
D: mm

(Audio-recorded consultation in general practice, GP7P24)

Two pieces of evidence demonstrate that the participants have agreed this is to be a new consultation. First, before the doctor used 'What can I do for you today?', he cleared the ground by establishing that there was nothing pending from previous consultations (lines 3–4). Second, in responding to the doctor's elicitor, the patient went to great lengths to contextualize the reason for his visit. He did this presumably because he could not assume the doctor to be already aware of it. Similar observations have been made in Finnish and US studies of consultations by Ruusuvuori (2000; 2005) and Heritage and Robinson (2006) respectively.

As we have said above, the distinction between new consultation vs. follow-up consultation, and the corresponding distribution of first concern elicitors, is only a scheme of interpretation. This means that, in actual consultations, participants use this distinction in a variety of ways and in order to accomplish a variety of functions. Consider Extract 2 again. As we have seen, the pragmatic approach is unable to analyse the patient's talk in line 2. However, if the patient's talk is looked at in its sequential environment and in the light of what we know about the opening sequence in general practice consultations, the patient's contribution becomes obvious. In line 1, the doctor defines the consultation as a new one. In line 2, the patient corrects the doctor's interpretation by reminding him of the reason why he has come ('... my blood test ...'). In line 3, the doctor acknowledges the repair and, together, the participants agree on the definition of this as a follow-up consultation.

What, then, does patient participation mean at the level of the opening sequence? As the discussion above makes it clear, in the opening sequence, patients do not just provide information. They also participate by contributing effectively to the definition of the consultation as a follow-up or as a new consultation. Since the use of first concern elicitors is a 'discourse strategy' (Gumperz 1982) and since the use of a first concern elicitor is 'best understood as a proposal made by the doctor to the patient as to how to view their interaction' (Gafaranga and Britten 2005: 85), patient participation means contributing to this negotiation, by confirming or correcting the doctor's understanding.

Briefly, the approach we have adopted here views patient participation as taking place not at the level of the consultation as a whole, but at the level of significant interactional activities. In other words, patients participate in the consultation by contributing to interactionally significant activities such as the opening of the consultation or formulation. It follows from this that, to understand patient participation, one starts by describing significant interactional activities and then proceeds to ask the question: what could patient participation mean in this activity, given what we know about it? It also follows that, as the list of significant conversational activities is an open-ended one, a conversation analytic perspective is unable to provide any 'definitive answer' to the question: what is patient participation? Instead, understanding patient participation must be seen as an ongoing project.

Improving patients' participation

In the introduction to this chapter, we noted that, at the policy level, there is a renewed emphasis on improving patient participation at the community level as well as at the level of the consultation. How to improve patient participation at the level of the consultation remains something of a mystery. Undertaken under the name of 'patient training', efforts to improve patient participation in the consultation do not seem to have borne expected results. For example, as Cegala et al. (2000: 210) report with reference to question asking, the results of studies of patient communication skills training 'have been inconsistent, with some research showing that trained patients ask more questions than untrained patients . . . and other studies reporting no significant difference in question asking between trained and untrained patients'. Even more worrying is Houtkoop's (1986) observation regarding formulation. Houtkoop shows that the strategy of training professionals to use formulation as a way of checking understanding may backfire because, in actual interaction, there is a preference for agreement after a formulation (Houtkoop 1986; Gafaranga and

Britten 2004). Likewise, training patients to use formulation might turn out to be unsuccessful because of the same preference. In our view, there are two explanations for this situation. First of all, patients' activities in the consultation have not been sufficiently understood for, as we have seen, little research has so far focused on *patients'* contributions in the consultation. Second, patient training, as practised in experimental projects, underestimates the normative nature of interactional activities. Thus, in the following, we briefly comment on the contribution an interactional activities perspective on patient participation, as illustrated in this chapter, can make to the question of how to improve patient participation.

Richards (2005) has identified two possible ways of conceptualizing the use of conversation analytic findings: 'discovery → prescription' versus 'description → informed action'. In the 'discovery – prescription' framework, once an interactional regularity has been described, people could be trained to use it. This seems to be the idea behind current efforts towards patients' communication skills training. For example, as indicated above, observation has revealed that other-formulating summaries are effective strategies for revealing one's understanding and, therefore, for checking understanding. Presumably, then, in order to improve patient participation, patients could be trained to use this strategy. However, the effectiveness of such training remains a rather controversial issue (see above). On the other hand, according to the 'description → informed action' professional practice framework, the findings of sequentially based analyses of interaction can be used to raise awareness. As Richards (2005: 6) puts it, 'By thinking in terms of raising awareness, directing attention, developing sensitivity and challenging assumptions, CA can contribute to informed professional action, helping professionals to deepen their understanding and develop new competencies.'

Although Richards' comment is phrased in terms of the training of professionals (health professionals in the present case), there is no doubt that it could apply to the training of patients as well. That is, CA findings could be used to raise patients' awareness of interactional phenomena. For example, patients could be made aware of the various functions of formulation, of the variations on the opening sequence and of how they can contribute, with the hope that improved participation would follow from improved awareness. Clearly, raising awareness is quite different from using prescriptive models for the purposes of teaching, for example the model of patient centredness described by Stewart et al. (1995).

Conclusion

Over the last few years, health policies have emphasized the participation of communities and patients in the provision of care. In the UK, these policies have translated into initiatives such as Patient Advice and Liaison services (PALs) and the Commission for Public and Patient Involvement in Health. However, while participation at the community level is relatively well defined, exactly what patient participation means at the level of the consultation remains unclear.

Our proposal is that CA can be a useful methodology for understanding patient participation in the consultation. The methodology we are proposing would consist of two stages. First, a conversational activity is described in order to understand it in detail. Second, once a detailed description of an interactional activity is available, we ask the question: what might patient participation mean here? By way of illustrating this methodology, we have looked at two interactional objects we have already described elsewhere, namely, formulation and the opening sequence in general practice consultations. When we raised the above question in the light of what we know about these interactional activities, it became clear that patient participation is multifaceted and that it varies depending on the interactional activity participants are involved in. Two conclusions were drawn from this observation. The first conclusion was that, in order to understand patient participation, one must look, not at the consultation as a whole, but rather at specific significant activities. Second, and following on from this, we concluded that from a CA perspective, there cannot be an overall answer to the question: what is patient participation? This is so because, in any interaction and at every stage 'both (or all) participants are contributing in some form or other' (Britten 2003). Rather, understanding patient participation must be seen as an ongoing project.

Finally, we looked at the question of improving patient participation. We respecified the question as one of understanding how CA findings about patient participation can be used. Since conversational structures are at the same time 'occasioned' and 'normative', along with Richards (2005), we concluded that a 'discovery – prescription' model would be futile. Rather, we argued that a 'description – informed action' model should be adopted. In this model, CA findings would be used to raise patients' and doctors' awareness of what patient participation in relevant conversational activities means (and see the Educational Supplement, p. 207).

Recommendations: summary

- Patient participation must be understood in terms of activities (e.g. seeking information) rather than in terms of linguistic forms (e.g. questions) for there is no necessary link between linguistic forms and pragmatic functions.
- In order to understand patient participation, the analyst must look at specific significant sequences.

- A CA perspective reveals that patient participation is multi-faceted and varies depending on the type of sequence. For example, participation in formulation is different from participation in the opening sequence.
- Understanding patient participation, from a CA perspective, must be seen as an ongoing project.
- CA findings can be used to raise health professionals' and patients' awareness of what patient participation in relevant conversational activities means, rather than to prescribe particular courses of action.

7 What is patient participation?

Reflections arising from the study of general practice, homoeopathy and psychoanalysis

Anssi Peräkylä, Johanna Ruusuvuori and Pirjo Lindfors

Commentary

This chapter continues the presentation of conversation analytic insights into patient participation, begun in Chapters 5 and 6. The focus of this chapter moves beyond the consultation's opening phase, and the activity of formulations, to explore the details of patient participation in relation to diagnostic and treatment phases in three different types of consultation.

The analyses centre on the following activities and types of consultation: (1) delivery and reception of diagnosis in general practice; (2) the delivery of treatment decisions in homoeopathy; and (3) the reception of interpretations in psychoanalysis. The analyses show that, in general practice consultations, the patient often remains silent after the doctor has delivered the diagnosis, and only comments in non-routine cases. In homoeopathy, practitioners provide varying amounts of space for the patient's comments in the treatment proposal. In psychoanalysis, practitioners actively pursue patients' comments to their interpretations.

Further to the illustration of different forms of patient participation across different consultation situations, the analyses also show that, in relation to each of the situations studied, there are alternative designs to professionals' turns at talk; one participatory, one non-participatory. Thus the particular consultation activities studied here highlight how the possible forms of patient participation are governed by the health professional's initial actions.

Beyond the specific findings it presents, this chapter also serves as an experiment in comparison. The data presented are from Finnish consultations in three clinical settings, and the analyses invite certain questions about patient participation and what it may be taken to mean in any given context.

By taking these Finnish data, the UK data presented elsewhere in this book, and the reader's own experiences as a starting point, we may want to consider, in future research, the influences of linguistic and cultural differences on the possible forms of participation for patients.

In a strict conversation analytic (CA) sense, participation includes all forms of action or omission of action in which an interactant is involved. In this sense, you could say that 'you cannot not participate' – just as Bateson (1972) said about communication 'you cannot not communicate'. The patient is inevitably participating in all health care encounters – by being bodily present, by using gaze, and by talking in any form. However, we will start with a different and more specific understanding of participation. We will talk about participation as the potential for patients to take part in key activities in three different types of health care encounter. Thus participation, as it is understood here, involves the ways in which patients are given opportunities to contribute to the discussion on *what the health problem is* and *what should be done about it*. See the Educational Supplement, pp. 207–8, for related heterial and exercises.

We approach this form of patient participation by presenting some of our observations concerning general practice, homoeopathy and psychoanalysis. The question of participation presents itself in a different way in each of these three types of service encounters, depending on the main task in hand. We will not be able to give an overall picture of patient participation in these three settings. Instead, we focus on one key activity in each that is essential in terms of the purpose of the consultation. In general practice, we examine the delivery and reception of diagnosis, in homoeopathy, we study the delivery and reception of treatment proposals and in psychoanalysis we analyse the reception of interpretations.

The data comprise 100 video-recorded and transcribed general practice consultations with 14 physicians, 40 homoeopathic consultations with five homoeopaths, and 58 audio-recordings of psychoanalytical sessions with three analysts.[1] The original data were recorded in Finnish.

Patient participation in the delivery and reception of diagnosis in general practice

Non-participatory diagnosis

In general practice consultations, diagnosis forms a central part of the general goal of alleviating patients' health-related problems. In the Finnish data of 71 diagnostic statements, two distinctively different trajectories in the delivery and reception of diagnosis can be found (and see Peräkylä 1998; 2002; 2006). One of them involves only minimal patient participation, whereas in the other, the patient is more active. In the 'non-participatory' trajectory, the diagnosis is preceded by a medical examination that is straightforward and routine, involving simple actions such as listening to the lungs of the patient or looking at X-ray pictures. This is followed by the delivery of diagnosis designed as a simple declarative statement, 'plain assertion'. The diagnosis is received by the patient staying silent or producing a minimal acknowledgement token (such as 'yeah' or in Finnish *joo*) (cf. Heath 1992). A move to discussion of treatment, or other future action, ensues. Extract 1 is one such case:

Extract 1 (D = doctor; P = patient)

D: (.hhh) Then the other dear had been a lit- >sorry the< ear
had been a little (0.3) reddish [the] ((looking at papers))
P: [↑YE]AH:.=
D: =nurse told ↑let's look at that too.
(0.5) ((Dr takes the instruments from the table))
P: Yeah:: it was this right e°ar°. .hh I do have
tried to bear it and then one gets those,
(12.0) ((Dr. looks into the ear))
D: There's still an infection in the
auditory canal.=I'll prescribe (.) °kind of° (.)
drops °for it°.
P: I've here this [kind of ones which I got, ((hand in pocket))
D: [I see

(Video-recorded consultation in general practice, Dgn 96 46B1)

The diagnosis (line 9–10: 'There's still an infection in the auditory canal') is preceded by a simple examination, as the doctor looks into the patient's ear. The direction from which the diagnostic evidence comes is clear: the patient cannot avoid knowing that the doctor was looking in his ear. The diagnosis is not contested by the patient, and the doctor does not in any way show anticipation of it becoming contested. There is no uncertainty involved.

In our data in general, and in this case in particular, these features of the interaction preceding the diagnosis were associated with 'plain assertion' delivery (the design of the diagnostic statement as a simple declarative statement) and the patient's passivity in receiving the diagnosis. In this particular case, the patient does not say anything in response to the diagnostic statement; his comment in line 12 concerns the treatment. Nor does the doctor show any orientation to the possibility of the patient talking about the diagnosis: in fact, he 'rushes' to the talk about prescription in line 10, thereby not leaving space for the patient to comment.

Participatory diagnosis

The 'participatory' diagnosis is usually preceded by a medical examination that is non-routine or problematic. This kind of examination can involve manifest uncertainty concerning the nature of the ailment, or discrepancy between the view expressed by the patient during the examination, and the actual diagnosis. Or alternatively, the examination can just be long and complicated. In such cases, the doctor often verbally refers to the evidence of the diagnosis, either explicitly or indirectly, and in response, patients may offer their comments. As a result, the progression of the consultation is halted, as the doctor cannot move directly to the discussion on future action. Extract 2 is a case in point:

Extract 2

```
D:  Well (.) we'll have to follow up how this thigh of
    yours, (0.6). hh begins to respond and, (0.8) it has
    indeed now clearly improved from °what
    it is[and,°
P:        [It has at least in terms of pain th[e:n.
D:                                             [Yeah:.
    (0.4)
D:  Yes:. .h >Did you have laboratory tests< now: sti[ll
P:                                                   [NO:.
    ((Ten lines omitted: talk about the timing of the tests))
D:  Yes:.
    (2.0)
D:  .hh Well (0.8) I haven:'t (0.2) I I (1.0) haven't
    (0.3) considered it as a (0.2) thrombosis.
P:  Mm hm,
D:  I think it isn't, (0.5) it would have,=if there would
    have been a beginning of a thrombosis then it would
    have been much more pain↑ful.
P:  Yes right.
D:  So certainly there are the VARICOSE veins.
    (0.8)
P:  Somethi- yeah I can feel the very lumps there
    in a certain position and when one tightens it,. hh
    then they appear quite here in the side so that. hh
    it is really like (.) one could s[ay a bumpy
D:                                   [Yeah:,
P:  road. (.) Eh bumps on a road ha ha[.hh
D:                                    [Yes.
```

(Video-recorded consultation in general practice, Dgn 3 1B2)

Here, the doctor explicitly rejects the diagnostic suggestion offered by the patient. The patient suffered from intense pain in her leg and was making a follow-up visit after sick leave. Early in the medical interview (data omitted for reasons of space), the patient suggested that the pain in her thigh might have been caused by exertion or by 'something either coming or going' in the thigh. The doctor treats this comment as referring to 'thrombosis', a diagnosis that the doctor subsequently rejects in her diagnostic utterance.

The rejection of the patient's diagnostic proposal is first delivered in lines 22–3. Then, in line 25, after a neutral acknowledgment by the patient, the doctor renews the rejection. After this, she explicates evidence that supports her conclusion. A thrombosis would have been more painful. Another, less serious diagnosis, varicose veins, framed as certain but also as one that might not exhaustively explain the patient's problems, is offered in line 29. After a brief interval, the patient in lines 31–6 tells the doctor about her own observations that support the diagnosis of varicose veins.

Thus, in Extract 2, a problematic or non-routine examination (which involved a degree of controversy and uncertainty) preceded a diagnostic statement that was couched with explication of evidence by the doctor, and the patient subsequently took part in discussing the diagnosis.

To summarize, in diagnosis, minimal patient participation in routine cases does not surface in the interaction as a problem, either for the patient or the doctor. In such cases, doctors do not invite the patient to participate, and patients do not actively offer their contributions. Patient participation is, however, relevant in the non-routine cases.

In the non-routine cases, we can then ask what the patient participation leads to. Roughly, a distinction can be made between cases where the patient's extended response to the diagnosis is consequential for the unfolding of the consultation, and cases where it is not. The response is consequential if the doctor takes up the patient's remarks concerning the diagnosis, for example, by returning to the medical interview or the physical examination. In our data, there are cases of both kinds (for more details, see Peräkylä 2002).

As a whole, the doctor possibly faces two choices in terms of patient participation in the diagnostic sequences. The first choice is whether or not to design the diagnosis in such a way that encourages more than a minimal response from the patient. As we have tried to show elsewhere (Peräkylä 1998; 2002), making explicit references to diagnosis is one way of encouraging that response. The second choice is what to do with the patient response: whether or not to topicalize it, whether or not to allow it to influence the unfolding of the consultation.

Patient participation in the delivery of treatment decisions in homoeopathy

Homoeopathy is a form of healing that relies on holistic principles – remedies are prescribed according to the totality of the person's physical, emotional and mental symptoms (Vithoulkas 1980; Chappell and Andrews 1996). The cornerstone of homoeopathic healing is to match the patient's reported symptoms to the codified descriptions of homoeopathic remedies in books such as *Materia Medica and Repertory* (Boericke et al. 1990). The aim is to find an individual treatment for the patient. Unlike in general practice consultations, actual diagnoses are not given but the treatment decision in itself implies the diagnosis. Medical tests or physical examination are usually not used: the treatment decision is preceded by and based upon an extensive verbal examination of the patient (for comparisons of homoeopathic and general practice consultations, see also Chatwin et al., Chapter 5 in this volume; Lindfors and Raevaara 2005; Ruusuvuori 2005).

In analysing the delivery and reception of treatment decisions in homoeopathic consultations, we concentrated on the extent to which the homoeopath offers or provides places for the patient to make verbal contributions related to the decision-making process (and see Lindfors 2005). In all 78 sequences of treatment discussion in the data, the treatment decision was either made or suggested by the homoeopath. Unlike in the diagnostic statements in general practice, some grounds for the decision were always integrated in its verbal formulation. In this sense, all patients were provided with at least some resources for commenting upon the homoeopath's decision. However, there were differences in the extent to which patients were involved in the decision-making process. In the first type of trajectory, the homoeopaths gave the treatment decision, waited for the patients' reply and continued with a new activity. In the second trajectory, the homoeopaths involved the patients by asking them to confirm their own perception about the present state of the healing process before announcing the treatment decision. In the third type of trajectory, patients were offered resources to agree or disagree with the upcoming treatment decision by giving either vocal or textual information concerning a potential match between their symptoms and the suggested homoeopathic symptom description. In all trajectories, patients' responses to the treatment decision were treated as relevant, but there was variation in the extent to which patients' agreement with the decision was pursued.

The following three extracts illustrate these different trajectories. In the first two, the proposal for treatment is given as the homoeopath's unilateral informing. However, there are differences between the two, regarding how the evidence for the proposal is explicated, and thus how the proposal is made available for the patient to comment upon. We have called these two types of decision-making non-participatory. In the last extract the way in which the proposal is delivered clearly makes it relevant for the patient to show her agreement or disagreement with the decision. This type of decision-making we have named participatory.

Non-participatory decision-making

Extract 3 shows a case where the treatment proposal is given as a 'plain' informing by the homoeopath. In line 1, the homoeopath says 'right' after reading her book. Thus she closes the previous activity and starts the treatment discussion by reporting her choice of remedy (lines 1–5):

Extract 3 (H = homoeopath; P = patient)

```
        (18.0) ((homoeopath looks at her books))
   H    .mt ↑right (0.4) I'll give you homoeopathic
        be:lladon°na°, (0.3) rarely used for skin skin symp-
        ((H looks at P, P nods))
        for ski::n use- ↑skin (1.0) nuture (0.2) hu- (2.0)
        used for skin problems, =but now it feels that in any case we
        will start with °it°. ((H looks down and arranges her
        papers))
        (0.8) ((P nods))
   H:   or I'll also give you sulphuris to begin with
        (0.2) so the sequela of cortisone (.) nuture (1.2)
        would go away and clean it up. ((H looks up to P))
        (1.2) ((P nods))
   P:   °mm:°
        (29.0) ((H looks at her books))
```

(Video-recorded consultation in homoeopathy, 13.1)

In lines 1–6, the homoeopath delivers her decision 'unilaterally' (see Collins et. al. 2005). The decision is designed as already made ('I'll give you') and not as something they should discuss together, even if there are features that mark it as tentative ('it feels that', line 5). The evidence for the decision is embedded in the informing. In lines 2–6, the homoeopath states that even though this remedy is rarely used for skin problems, it would be the right choice in this case. In this way she implies that the decision is based on the individual characteristic of this patient's problem.

In lines 9–11, the homoeopath informs the patient about another medication she will be given for her rash. Just as with the previous decision, this one also is designed as definitive. The patient acknowledges the decisions by nodding (lines 3, 8 and 12) and by saying '°mm:°' (line 13). The patient's acknowledgements could be interpreted as mere receipts of the information given, or alternatively as containing an element of agreement with the decision. In any case, the homoeopath treats the patient's responses as sufficient to move on to another activity.

In Extract 4, the treatment proposal is also presented definitively (lines 64–66, 69–70). However, unlike in the previous extract, the chain of reasoning leading to the decision is made explicit, and the patient's viewpoint is integrated in the reasoning:

Extract 4

```
 1  P:  [(but in any case, yes but in any case)
 2      the kind of whole situation (0.2) is better.
 3      (.)
 4  H:  ye[s.
 5  P:    [so if it can't (.) it can't be thought about as
 6      a period of an hour or even a day >so if< you think about a
 7      one-week-period °so°,
 8      (0.2)
 9  H:  of[cour°se.°
10  P:    [it's better.=
11  H:  =right.
12      (0.4)
13  H:  t'and (.) if: (.) we then think about this whole thing now
14      you: (.) last spring we started erm, (2.8)
15      your (1.0) .ng hhhh the sixteenth of June (.) ((H looks at
16      notes)) [(you visited)] here the first[(time)]
17  P:          [yes .        ]               [yes.  ]
18      (.)
19  H:  right, (1.0) mt at that time you've had s:- weakness
20      in your hand quite a lot andh, (2.0) diplo↑pia
21      almost every day. (0.2)
22  H:  [or  ] every now and then
23  P:  [Mm:.]
24      (3.6) ((H reads her notes))
25  H:  anyway this has like all the time little by little
26      (0.8) got better now then.
27      (.)
28  P:  yes it has.
        ((7 lines omitted, P talks about his hand that has healed))
36  H:  =yes, and it was that phosphorus which was such[that
37  P:                                                  [it (.)
38  H:  helped.)]
39  P:  it felt  ] good[the  ]nh.
40  H:                 [mm.  ]
```

(0.6) ((H looks at her notes))
H: righ:t. (.) mt .hhh well t- (.) even this kind of thing can
happen then so like this that (.) the: (.) old ailment can
in a way get worse=> we call it the first reaction?
(0.2)
P: [right,
H: [and they are not so dangerous but typically sort of
(.) temporary as: (0.6) now in this case here and
.hh it was that actually the eczema in the summer it
was a sort of a first reaction as well,
(.)
P: yes.
(.)
H: and they are then like connected with (.) this kind of
recovery: (.) process,
(1.0)
H: which is followed up then.=but now as this was this kind of
substance with high potency so (0.6) let's think/we'll
think that the effect of this one would last longer,
((H looks at P)) (.) ((P nods))
H: so now we won't do anything at all actually but
wait for a month to see how far >this then<
this (0.6) recovery process continues.
P: *jooh.* ((complying response particle in Finnish))
(.)
H: and then if it stops (.) so only then we'll renew
this dose.
(.)
P: *joo.* ((P nods))
(0.4)
H: so that's the way we'll (.) go ahead now andh,
((H moves on to another topic))

(Video-recorded consultation in homoeopathy, 5.2)

In this extract, the homoeopath works to reach a shared understanding of the patient's present state of health and of the effects of previous medication before proposing future treatment. She does this with the help of summarizing evaluations (lines 25–6, 36–38) and understanding checks which call for the patient's confirmation (lines 14–16, 21–22, 36–38). Thus, she aligns with the patient's preceding positive evaluation of his state of health (1–2, 5–7, 10) and also upgrades the evaluation to accommodate the whole healing process and the remedy that has helped. Once she has received the patient's confirmation, she proceeds to give an explanation for the symptoms the patient has mentioned earlier as problematic (42–57). She integrates this explanation with the grounds that she gives (lines 57–60) for her treatment proposal that follows (lines 61–63, 66–67).

Thus, in this case, the homoeopath makes explicit the chain of reasoning leading to her decision, and attaches this reasoning to the patient's own evaluation of his state of health. She also works to attain a shared understanding of the patient's present condition before suggesting further treatment (and see Maynard 1992). Even though the actual proposal is given as definitive, the homoeopath treats the patient's own evaluation of his condition and the helpful remedy as relevant, and thus enhances patient participation.

A further look at the consultation shows that the patient receives the decision with a complying *joo*-particle (lines 64 and 69) (see Sorjonen 2001).[2] The *joo*-particle in line 64 is given immediately, and the one in line 69 almost immediately, after the homoeopath's decision: there are no signs of treating it as problematic (Pomerantz 1984). Both *joo*s end with a falling terminal contour, indicating that the patient will not continue his turn. The patient also nods with his latter *joo*-response. Even after this there is space for the patient to topicalize the decision, but the patient does not use this possibility. These features, together with earlier research by Sorjonen on *joo* as a proposal of compliance in this context, indicate that the patient treats the homoeopath's decision as acceptable.

Participatory decision-making

In the next extract (5), the patient's agreement with the homoeopath's treatment decision is explicitly pursued, and the patient is offered resources to form an independent opinion about the suggested remedy. Just before the extract the homoeopath has said that she is about to refer to a book to check the description of a remedy called caliumcarbonicum. The homoeopath gives the patient the homoeopathic book to read and to consider if the remedy under scrutiny matches her symptoms. The homoeopath also gives instructions to the patient on where she should start reading:

Extract 5

```
H:   I'll: let you readh. ((H gives the book to P))
P:   ↑o↓kay.
     (2.0) ((P picks up the book))
H:   have a look<
     (1.0)
P:   in there.
H:   ye::s.
```

((127 lines omitted, P reads and topicalizes symptom descriptions in relation to her own symptoms))
152 (11.0) ((both are reading))
153 P: mm ↑mm, anxiety, (0.2) appears?, (1.5) around the
154 upper middle of the abdomen ye:s, >this is the place
155 where that cramp always appears when I'm uneasy.
156 (3.0)
157 H: hh hh
158 (1.0)
159 P: this does match quite nice[ly.
160 H: [mm.
((10 lines omitted, H talks about the benefit of P reading the book herself))
171 P: .mt I'm not afraid of being alone nor dark- darkness
172 nor ghosts but high places scare the hell out of me.
173 H: *.hnii.* ((Finnish dialogue particle))
174 (4.0) ((P reads and H writes down))
175 P: that's not mentioned here.
176 H: mm mm?,
177 (3.0) ((P reads and H writes down))
178 P: but it doesn't have to cover everything.
179 (13.0) ((P reads and H writes down))
180 P: yeah a lot of them are in here yeah?;
181 (0.5)
182 P: ↑oh ↓ho.
183 (1.0)
184 P: even arthritis that's right.
185 H: mm.
186 (1.0)
187 P: pain::: (.) from exercising.
188 (2.0)
189 P: numbness ye:s.
190 (0.8)
191 P: quite ↑well.
192 (2.0)
193 P: .snff it matches.
((P continues reading))
194 H: ↑yes::.
195 (1.0)
196 H: [let's put it in a bag.
197 P: [( ) ( )
198 P: *joo.* .hh h h

(Video-recorded consultation in homoeopathy, 33)

The homoeopath gives the homoeopathic book to the patient (line 18) so the patient may check for herself whether her symptoms match with the suggested remedy. On receiving the book the patient takes an active role in searching for matches between her symptoms and the description in the book (e.g. lines 153–4, 171–2). She also produces explicit evaluations of how well the suggested descriptions match with her symptoms (line 159). She observes something lacking from the description of the book (line 175) but evaluates this as not a problem (line 178). Between lines 180–93 the patient points out the 'good match' between the book and her symptoms. In this way, she displays agreement with the homoeopath's treatment suggestion. Following this, in line 196 the homoeopath makes the final decision, saying 'let's put it in a bag', and the patient complies.

This extract contains participatory elements in that the homoeopath works to get the patient's compliance with her suggestion, by providing the patient with resources for arriving at the same conclusion. However, as in the other extracts (as well as in the whole data), the actual decision is made or suggested by the homoeopath. Thus, the question remains as to whether one type of procedure described above offers the patient better chances to take part in the actual decision-making than any of the others. Do any of these procedures make it easier for the patient to reject the proposal offered, for example? On the other hand, the procedures of the homoeopaths do seem to differ in the ways in which they make explicit the grounds of the decision to the patient, and in the extent to which they treat as relevant the attainment of shared understanding of these grounds with the patient. Thus, the different degrees of participation in the treatment proposals in homoeopathy seem to have more to do with working towards the patients' affiliation and compliance with the homoeopath's decision than with opportunities to take part in the actual decision-making.

Patient participation in the reception of interpretations in psychoanalysis

Psychoanalysis is a very particular type of patient–provider encounter. In psychoanalysis, the patient explores his or her mind and relations to significant others, with the aim of increasing his or her self-understanding and hence alleviating suffering. Psychoanalytic treatment involves frequent (three to four per week) sessions during which the patient talks freely about his or her life while the analyst listens and sometimes intervenes with questions or comments.

Interpretations are particular types of interventions in psychoanalysis. They are the analyst's statements about the patient's mind. They are meant to help the patient to see and understand unconscious aspects of his or her experience and behaviour (Greenson 1967: 39–45; Rycroft 1995: 85).

Interpretations are usually devised by the analyst using verbal material that the patient has produced in the analytic sessions. In a broad sense, most interpretations involve rearrangement of the elements of the patient's narratives. In the interpretations, the analyst connects, highlights and re-contextualizes what the patient has said during the analytic hour. In this sense, interpretations involve a particular form of patient participation: they are largely made up of the materials that the patient has brought to the analyst.

In this chapter, however, we will be looking at the patient's *responses* to the interpretations.

Non-participatory cases

Patients' responses to interpretations can be divided into three broad classes; different classes of responses regularly occur in the same sequence. Sometimes patients produce *acknowledgement tokens* such as 'Mm' or 'Yeah': responses that are similar to those that patients most often give after hearing the diagnosis in general practice (see above). However, cases where such tokens constitute the patient's sole response to an interpretation are very rare. The patients can also respond to interpretations by *expressing their attitude towards the interpretation in a compact form*. This can involve outright rejection (for example, 'I̲ don't think the rules were that strict'), displays of scepticism (for example, 'Y̲eah who knows,') displays of commitment to 'mental processing' of the interpretation, without clearly agreeing or disagreeing with it (for example, 'Wonder if it could be like tha̲t,'), or agreement (for example, 'It is absolutely true'). In more than half of cases in our data, the patients end up talking even more extensively about the interpretations. They take up some aspect of the interpretation and continue discussion on it, by illustrating or explaining what was proposed by the analyst. Peräkylä (2006) has called these responses *elaborations of the interpretation*. Elaborations convey agreement with and understanding of the interpretation. They are often preceded by other types of responses: the patient may first respond to an interpretation with an acknowledgement token and/or with a compact expression of attitude, and move thereafter to an elaboration.

We have argued elsewhere (Peräkylä 2005) that analysts and patients orient to elaborations as the kind of response that the interpretations seek. For the analysts' part, this orientation is revealed in their actions that follow type one (minimal acknowledgement tokens) and type two (compact expressions of attitude) responses. After such responses, analysts regularly either remain silent, invite patients to say what is in their mind, or add new elements to the interpretation, thus creating a new opportunity for the patient to respond. In other words, analysts actively seek patients' participation that goes beyond mere acknowledgement or acceptance/rejection of the interpretation.

Sometimes a similar orientation becomes manifest in the patient's conduct. Extract 6 is an example. Prior to the interpretation, the analyst has pointed out that no intense feelings appear in the patient's talk. In the interpretation (only the final part is shown here) she proposes that the patient somehow 'empties her mind' during the psychoanalytic sessions. The patient responds only minimally to the analyst's interpretation in line 11. After a silence of 8 seconds, the analyst formulates the patient's action as problem-indicative by saying 'You don't sound excited'. This formulation invites an account from the patient for her (minimal) recipient action *vis-à-vis* the interpretation. In response to the formulation, the patient puts into words her orientation to a 'duty' to produce talk that is linked to the interpretation (lines 15–19).

Extract 6 (A = analyst; P = patient)

```
A:   .mth So that it will never be allowed to be
     examined it. hhh it will never be like
     allowed to examine to be examined and then it will not not
     be possible .hhh #erm# to eh >#nomehow< (0.5) ehhh#
     learn to know it or: or somehow (.) .mthh
P:   mhhhhhhhh
A:   or #in that way to increase <your some kind of
     (0.5) integrity or># (.) (.) something whatever
     it would then <be>.
     (0.4)
P:   Mmm,
     (8.0)
A:   .hh You don't sound ex°ited°.
     (0.7)
P:   mhha [ha I'm desperately trying to find something
A:        [hhe heh he
P:   #to say# .h[hhhh that that could
A:              [.hhhh Mm mm,
P:   be c(h)onnected to [this.
A:                      [mhhe
P?:   .hhhh
     (0.3)
```

Thus, in Extract 6, both parties put into words an expectation that the patient expresses her views concerning the interpretation through something more than a minimal acknowledgement. The analyst's formulation in line 13 invites an account from the patient, and in her account, the patient shows her orientation to an obligation to talk about the interpretation.

Participatory cases

As pointed out above, in more than half of the cases the interpretations lead to the patient taking up and elaborating what was proposed by the analyst. In elaborations, patients' participation in interpretation is at its fullest, as it were: the patient takes up the interpretation and continues it by adopting the perspective that was suggested in the interpretation, in relation to the objects of his/her life. Extract 7 is an example of an elaboration. The analyst proposes in his interpretation that the patient's experience of a rival colleague who is currently in trouble in her profession, is linked to the patient's experience of her siblings who were ill, and one of whom died, when the patient was a child. In Extract 7, the final part of the interpretation is shown:

Extract 7

A: so there's also that similarity that when (1.0)
Aino is in trouble, (0.6) so she's like ill.
(1.6)
A: A bit like she was about to die.
(1.2)
A: (tch) And possibly will °die° .in her profession.
(3.0)
A: So then it is difficult, (0.8) really to be angry
enough at her, (0.6) as you feel sympathy °for her°.
P: .mh (0.4) It is absolutely true.
(11.0)
P: .thh it is absolutely true that I feel sympathy.
(1.4)
?P: .nff
(2.6)
A: So: it is >I think that< it is pretty close to the feeling
that (0.6) your ill sibl°ings° (0.4) °arose in you°.
P: Mm
(10.0)
P: .thh difficult to be angry.=difficult to compete.
=difficult to be env°ious.°
A: Y[eah.
[( )
(4.6)
P: What is there to be envious for when the other °is
laying down° (0.8) about to °die°.
(0.4)
A: Quite °right°.

(Audio-recorded consultation in psychoanalysis, AL11 811-985)

The patient's elaboration begins in line 20 (lines 10 and 12 involve agreement, and not elaboration). She first illustrates what was proposed by the analyst in the interpretation, with a list of the feelings with which she has difficulties. The first item basically repeats what was suggested by the analyst in an earlier part of the interpretation (difficult to be angry, lines 8–9). After that, the patient names two other feelings. The 'object' of these feelings is left unspecified: the patient seems to show that they are applicable both to the sister and to the colleague – thereby maintaining the linkage suggested by the analyst in his interpretation. After an agreement token by the analyst (line 22), the patient continues the elaboration by animating her childhood self considering her sick sister's situation (lines 25–6). Through her elaboration, the patient takes up the interpretation and eventually continues it in her own terms.

After the analyst has delivered an interpretation, and the patient has responded to it, there is a slot for the 'third position' action in which the analyst has an opportunity to act on the patient's elaboration or other response (the 'second position'). The directions taken by the analysts in these third position actions vary: sometimes they build upon the patient's elaboration (thereby treating the elaboration as an 'adequate' response to the initial interpretation) but in some cases, they may – for example, by returning to and pursuing the initial interpretation – indicate that the patient's response was not the one being sought by the analyst. Sometimes, in cases where the analyst's third position action builds upon the patient's elaboration, that third position action may instigate a cycle of collaborative description in which the patient, along with the analyst, participates in sketching an aspect of the patient's experience. Extract 8 is a case in point.

At the beginning of the extract, the patient is talking about her grief after the recent death of her partner. In examining her own feelings, she has realized that she is worried that she might get stuck in her grief. In line 18, the analyst begins an interpretation in which he makes a link between the patient's current difficulties in grieving, and her 'childhood sorrows'. After a minimal agreement token by the patient (line 22), the analyst adds an increment to the interpretation in which he points out that in her childhood, the patient felt that sorrows have to be 'left behind' quickly (lines 24–5). Finally, overlapping with the patient's turn beginning, the analyst adds a third component (line 28) which animates the patient's attitude:

Extract 8

```
01  P:   . . . maybe there is some kind of
02       fear that I . . .
         ((five lines omitted))
08  P:   or that I will become like  [that
09  A:                               [((coughs)) hmm
```

(.)
P: old relative of mine so I will just walk
around then and say oh I wish I could get away.
(1.0)
P: I mean that is no (.) .hhh .hh (0.3) way to live.
(0.4)
P: You either live or you ↓don't live.
(1.8)
A: .hhh I do think that it has (0.5) uh considerable
dimensions that thing so that it .hhh again I would indeed
connect it to your (0.4) childhood situations to these
(.) gre[at sorrows.
P: [Yeah:,
(0.3)
A: When >you have the kind of< feeling that they must just
(0.4) be left behind right °away°.
(0.5)
P: ye[:s (just<)
A: [One shouldn't be drawn in[to griev°ing°.
P: [To dance and to sing.
(.)
A: Yes,
P: So that others would be happy (.) and pleased with me.
(.)
A: Yes and you too would feel bet°ter°.
(2.3)
A: But there is the problem then that .hhh
how much of that grief then goes completely un°grieved°.
P: Yes well: now at this moment so far there's not any .hhh
.hhh KRÖHHHH (0.4) köh köh krhmm (0.4) mt .hhh
great danger yet that I would get rid of it.
(3.3)
P: But but I (0.5) well I balance things so that,
(1.0) go around (0.5) and do things and. (0.8) .hhh
I went to buy some bulbs of amaryllis and will put them
to the ground . . .

(Audio-recorded consultation in psychoanalysis, Tul4: 1, B18: 2-7)

The first part of the patient's elaboration of the interpretation is started by the word 'just' after the second agreement token in line 27, then aborted, and completed in line 29. The elaboration is sequentially tied to the second part of the analyst's interpretation (lines 24–5) in which he described the patient's childhood scene. The patient uses metaphorical language to illustrate the same experience that the analyst was describing: she moved on 'to dance and to sing', instead of allowing herself to take time for grieving. After an agreement token by the analyst (line 31), the patient expands her description of the childhood scene. She adds an explanatory dimension to the description, referring to the expectations of 'others' as a reason for her inability to mourn as a child (line 32).

The analyst's third position action begins in line 34. After an agreement token 'yes' (Finnish *nii*, which does affiliative work in this context, Sorjonen 2001), he produces an utterance that is designed as a grammatical continuation of the patient's preceding turn (line 32). Here, the analyst adds another reason for the patient's inability to mourn: by not mourning, the patient also made herself feel better. As a whole, the interpretation–elaboration–extension sequence accomplishes a momentary communion of minds. The analyst and the patient collaboratively draw a sketch of sensitive aspects of the patient's childhood experience. The analyst's extension utterance complements the patient's elaboration by offering a parallel reason for the patient's childhood mourning behaviour.

However, the analyst's extension also involves a shift in topical focus. The patient's version of the 'reasons for' her childhood behaviour of mourning focuses on *others*: she sees this pattern as socially induced. In his third position utterance, the analyst points out the inner dynamics of the patient's mind: getting rid of sorrows quickly, helped the patient, too. This may be important in terms of the psychotherapeutic process, as the analyst opens up a perspective for the patient to examine her *own* mind instead of explaining her behaviour through the expectations of others.

The patient does not verbally respond to the analyst's extension, and after a silence of 2.3 seconds (line 35), the analyst continues his third position action with an assessment (lines 36–7). He explicitly adopts a new perspective to what was described in the preceding talk, by pointing out that the patient's way of dealing with sorrows (described in the analyst's interpretation, the patient's elaboration, and the analyst's extension of it) has its drawbacks: grief remains unexpressed. Notably, the analyst adopts the generic present tense here, thus making his assessment applicable both to the patient's childhood situation and to her current grief. In her subsequent talk (lines 38–40), and in a somewhat sarcastic tone, the patient declines the relevancy of the proposal for her current situation. Thereafter she moves on to another topic (lines 42–5).

In sum, psychoanalytic interpretations invite active patient participation. They make relevant not only acknowledgement, agreement or disagreement by the patient, but also that he or she adopts the perspective proposed in the interpretation and applies it to further examination of his or her experience. This kind of patient response can be part of a dialogical process where the participants collaboratively construct a verbal description of the patient's mind.

Conclusion

In each of the three settings, the question of participation set itself differently according to the key activity for that particular encounter. In general practice, we analysed participatory and non-participatory trajectories of giving and receiving diagnosis; in homoeopathy, we described participatory and non-participatory ways to deliver the treatment decision; in psychoanalysis, we focused on the ways in which patients participate in the interpretations made by the analysts on the patients' preceding talk. In each setting, we located different ways in which, and degrees to which, participation was made relevant with regard to these activities. In general practice, the relevancy of patient participation varied according to the characteristics of the cases (routine vs. non-routine) and was initially invoked by the doctors according to how they designed the diagnosis. In homoeopathy, the relevancy of patient participation was tied to affiliating with the homoeopath's treatment decision and was concretized to different degrees by the homoeopath. In psychoanalysis, patient participation in analysts' interpretations was highly relevant for the key goal of the encounter: it ensured patient collaboration in exploring the patient's mind.

CA as a method is suitable for the analysis of distinct activities. It makes it possible to describe the trajectories through which key goals of a particular institutional encounter are realized. It can show what sorts of actions are treated as relevant by the participants in the realization of these activities. Through description of these participants' orientations, CA can explain how different structures and patterns of the activities analysed provide for different (blocking or enhancing) opportunities for patient participation. However, there are also limitations to what can be said about patient participation drawing upon CA and/or the analyses presented in this chapter.

In structural terms, all the activities explored in this chapter involve opportunities for patient participation *in second position*, i.e. in actions that are responsive to the professional's actions. In each setting, there are also *first position* acts that could and should be examined in terms of patient participation. They involve patients' *questions, requests for advice* (in homoeopathy), *patients' proposals for treatment* (in homoeopathy), *candidate diagnoses* (in medical consultations), and *stories* (in psychoanalysis). Further CA-informed study of these first position activities would be needed in order to form a broader picture of patient participation in each setting.

Another limitation is that, as such, CA does *not* offer tools for description of patient participation in the context of the whole consultation. In this article, we focused on patients' opportunities to take part in *distinct activities* (diagnosis in general practice, treatment proposals in homoeopathy, interpretations in psychoanalysis). These activities are recurrent and central in the three settings, but there are also other key activities in each setting. Therefore, our observations should not be read as an analysis of *all* patient participation in these settings (and see Chatwin et al., Chapter 5 in this volume; Gafaranga and Britten, Chapter 6 in this volume; Jones and Collins, Chapter 8 in this volume). However, we might want to discuss the possibilities of broadening the analysis by also studying the other main activities in each setting from this perspective (and see the Educational Supplement, pp. 207–8). We could ask whether it would be possible or desirable to develop a 'CA-informed' measure for patient participation in each different setting by combining the analyses of the different activities from this perspective.

However, even with the analyses of distinct activities, the following substantial points can be made. In each setting that we studied (or, more specifically, in each setting-specific activity), patient participation took a distinct form. The relevancy of these forms of patient participation ultimately arises from the overall goal of the encounter, as well as from the theory of healing that guides the interaction (see Peräkylä et al. 2005). The observed orientation of the homoeopaths to securing the patients' compliance with the treatment decision, for example, may originate with the necessity to rely exclusively on patients' reported symptoms. We might want to discuss, however, *whose* relevancies these are – the professionals', the patients', the relevancies of both, or the relevancies of the researcher?

Patient participation (in the activities that we have described) can be described in terms of 'more' or 'less' participation. In each setting, we made a distinction between cases where the patient participated 'more' and cases where the patient participated 'less'. Making comparisons regarding degrees of participation across each type of consultation, however, is analytically problematic. The activities studied are not entirely equivalent and the relevancy of participation is tied to the institutional goal of the encounter. Thus, a similar trajectory of action (e.g. when a professional integrates the grounds for his/her decision in the announcement to the patient) may seem more participatory in the context of delivering diagnosis in a general practice consultation than in making treatment decisions in homoeopathy.

Perhaps a better way to do a comparison is to look at the structure of setting-specific activities (diagnosis in general practice, treatment proposals in homoeopathy, and interpretations in psychoanalysis) regarding the amount of patient participation that is relevant in each. 'More than minimal' patient participation is *constitutive* in psychoanalytic interpretations as the interpretative sequence is treated as incomplete without such patient participation. In general practice, 'more than minimal' participation is *contingent:* whether or not it is relevant depends on specific circumstances related to the diagnostic sequence. In homoeopathy, participation is centred on the idea that patients should be given resources to understand and to agree with the decision. The orientation to 'more than minimal' participation, to pursuing the patient's compliance with the treatment decision, could be constitutive in two senses. On the one hand, it might be essential for the continuity of the treatment relationship and thus for the maintenance of the practice. On the other hand, it might be essential in terms of the holistic treatment ideology, where the recovery of the patient would require commitment to the suggested treatment.

Further, our analysis does *not* warrant the conclusion that 'more' participation (in the activities that we examined) is equal to a good or a successful encounter, and 'less' participation is equal to a bad or less successful encounter. The form and the amount of patient participation may be involved in the 'goodness' of an encounter, but in manifold ways. In general practice, for example, a good and successful diagnostic sequence may in many routine cases involve minimal patient participation. We might ask, to what extent is patient participation recommendable? Is it recommendable in any context? How does it affect professional authority?

In general practice, much of the patients' participation seems to be dependent on the way in which GPs design the diagnosis and on whether GPs take up patients' extended responses to diagnosis. Even though a patient's *joo* as a response to a GP's diagnosis or a homoeopath's treatment decision is compliant, it is also minimal. It implies that patients do not consider that they would need to give a more extensive display of compliancy in this context, regardless of whether or not they agree with the decision. We could then ask, whether the observation that *joo* is *treated* as a sufficient response to diagnosis or treatment decision gives grounds to claim that it *should* be sufficient. It has been shown (Stivers 2002) that in American medical consultations a plain confirmation is not treated by the doctors as a sufficient response to a treatment decision. This raises questions concerning whether this has to do with cultural or linguistic differences or perhaps with the specific characteristics of the activity in question. Whether the American practice is more participatory than the Finnish one remains to be seen.

We also need to bear in mind that 'more' patient participation in terms of verbal contributions is not equal to the patient's actual participation in clinical decision-making. In the homoeopathic consultations, the actual treatment decision is suggested and also made by the homoeopath. The homoeopath offers the patient opportunities to participate by making the grounds of the decision explicit and by treating the patient's consent as relevant. We could discuss whether this level of participation can make a difference from the patient's point of view. Is it enough that the patient's own stance towards the problem is treated as important, or that he or she is given an active role in testing and approving the professional's suggestion? On the other hand, we can ask whether patient participation can also be regarded as a form of persuasion, as a way to achieve certain professional goals. Or if it is really participation rather than another form of involvement, for example, consent.

Notes

1. The results presented here are from two research projects funded by the Academy of Finland.
2. According to Sorjonen, as a response to directives in Finnish, *joo* is a proposal of compliance while the alternative response particle *nii* treats the suggested course of action as possible, and this way foreshadows disagreement. The function of *joo* as proposing compliance is especially clear in cases when the directive is constructed as a 1st person plural imperative (as in the case above, where the Finnish version is 'Et nyt *ei* sitte oikeestaan *tehdä* yhtään mitään vaan *odotellaan*' 'ja sitten vasta *uusitaan* tää annos') (see Sorjonen 2001: 214–20, 257).

Recommendations: summary

- The significance of patient participation in terms of the purpose of the consultation varies in different types of encounters. Thus, recommendations concerning participation should always be considered in relation to the medical context in question.
- Before we can make recommendations about how to enhance patient participation, we need detailed descriptive analysis of the interactional consequences of each activity to which we refer.
- More verbal contributions by patients do not necessarily equate with more actual participation in the definition of the agenda or in the decision-making. In finding ways to enhance patient participation, attention must be paid to the *placement* of verbal contributions, both within a sequence of actions as well as in the context of the larger consultation activity (e.g. diagnosis, treatment discussion).

8 Nursing assessments and other tasks

Influences on participation in interactions between patients and nurses

Aled Jones and Sarah Collins

Commentary

The focus on nurses' communication with patients in this chapter offers a distinct contribution to the book, as well as a point of comparison. Three different types of nurse–patient encounter are considered: (1) hospital admission interviews; (2) diabetes review consultations in primary care; and (3) consultations in a hospital outpatients clinic for cancers of the head or neck.

The analyses focus on how the patient's contributions to these encounters are grounded in the ways in which the interview is organized and its topics prioritized through nurses' talk. Particular qualities of these encounters and their influence on patients' participation are identified. Two areas of influence are explored: (1) factors in the delivery of nursing care that restrict (or shape the possible form of) participation; and (2) practices that enhance participation.

In relation to factors that can be said to restrict patients' participation, the analyses show how, in nurses' communication with patients, topics can be defined and curtailed by the need to complete certain tasks, particularly those relating to documentation. At the same time, within the routine performances of nursing tasks, there are also opportunities for patients to comment in ways that display their particular concerns and understandings.

On the basis of our analyses and observations, we discuss some of the consequences of these nursing encounters for patient participation. Finally, we explore the implications of our findings for policy, practice, and education, and make suggestions for how patients' participation in nursing encounters may be promoted.

By drawing on other data, including interviews with nurses and doctors, this chapter brings into view connections across a patient's consultations with a range of health professionals. Thus, it begins to open out the discussion of contexts, levels, and a conceptual framework for studying patient participation in the concluding chapters in Part III.

Introduction

In all areas of nursing, the importance of involving patients in their care and communicating with them is emphasized. Nurses are often portrayed (and portray themselves) as the patient's advocate, for example, 'making [patients] feel that they are full partners. . . [and] establishing what their hopes and expectations are' (Nolan and Caddock 1996: 12).

These standards are not always realized. Observational research has shown nurses' communication with patients to be primarily task-related, running counter to a patient-centred view of patients as individuals requiring individual care. Much of nurses' communication with patients occurs during routine tasks, such as medication rounds (Macloed Clark 1983; Whittington and McLaughlin 2000); and while nursing staff express commitment to communication with patients, in practice, they may accord it low priority (Armstrong-Esther et al. 1994; Nolan et al. 1995).

The literature points to a number of reasons why this orientation to task predominates in interaction, and why communication opportunities are minimized, with patients' concerns remaining unexplored or undocumented. One constraint concerns the effects of patient records, templates and other forms of documentation on the interaction. Take, for example, the admissions interview, conducted on a patient's arrival in hospital. Barrett's (1988) study in an Australian psychiatric hospital described the process by which patients' detailed verbal accounts were reduced to sparse entries in written records, and their descriptions transformed into textbook views of the signs and symptoms of schizophrenia. In a UK-based ethnographic study of nursing care, Latimer (2000: 91) remarked that nurses conduct admission interviews as if looking at the patient 'according to a grid of perceptions and then noting according to a code'.

Another source of explanation concerns the role of nurses alongside doctors in the delivery of a patient's care. Nurses are often in the position of following on from, or supporting, a doctor's consultations with the same patient. This brings its own constraining influences (Williams 2000; Charles-Jones et al. 2003; Collins et al. 2003).

A third reason given for the emphasis on tasks over the communication with the patient is lack of time (Ashworth 1980; Bond 1983; Byrne and

Heyman 1997; Latimer 2000; Whittington and McLaughlin 2000), particularly in relation to acute care settings. Conversely, studies of community nursing (such as Sefi 1988; Hunt 1991; Adams 2001) have highlighted respects in which nurses' communication with patients and family members in their own homes is unhurried and centred on the individual.

All these factors – the task in hand, the roles and remits of the nurse, the time available, the particular health care setting – contribute to forms of patient participation in nurse consultations. In our own teaching, for example, we find that nurses frequently raise these constraints and their interrelation – the difficulties of consulting via templates (for example, in review consultations for patients with chronic illness); the responsibilities nurses incur in following on from, or preparing the ground for, doctors' communication with patients; and the lack of time for communicating and the difficulty of prioritizing it over other tasks, particularly perhaps on hospital wards.

The aim of this chapter is to explore, drawing on three different types of nurse–patient encounter in hospital and primary care settings, some consequences of the focus on task. With reference to recordings of nurse–patient interaction, the analyses highlight factors which shape the possible forms of patient participation, and show features of the communication that enhance it.

This chapter is organized as follows. An introduction to the data is first provided, followed by a description of the types of encounter studied, and of the tasks these encounters accomplish. The significance of these nursing encounters for patients' care is then discussed. The analysis is presented in two parts. The first part explores factors that restrict, or shape the possible form of, participation; the second part illustrates communication features that enhance patients' participation. A discussion of influences on patient participation follows and, finally, the conclusions are drawn.

Description of the data

The data comprise 49 video/audio-recorded nurse–patient encounters, in three different settings – 27 admissions interviews in a district general hospital, 19 review consultations for Type 2 diabetes in general practice, and three specialist cancer nurse consultations in a head and neck cancer outpatients' hospital clinic.

The participating nurses (36 in total) varied in their roles, responsibilities, and degree of specialization and autonomy. In the district general hospital admissions interviews, nurses ranged from staff nurse to ward manager. In the general practice diabetes review consultations, some nurses assisted the doctor, while others had almost complete responsibility for diabetes care. In the head and neck cancer clinic, one specialist cancer nurse took part.

Fifty-three patients were involved – 27 in the admissions interviews, 23 in the diabetes review consultations and three in the head and neck cancer clinic. In the hospital admissions interviews, patients with a range of ailments were being admitted into wards in acute medicine and surgery, neurology and coronary care. In the diabetes review consultations, patients had Type 2 diabetes (diagnosed 18 months to 12 years previously). In the head and neck cancer clinic, patients were attending for their first or second visit, during which the diagnosis was delivered and treatment was discussed.

Other data, collected in conjunction with these consultations, are employed to convey the broader scene within which these interactions are situated. These data include: doctor consultations for the same patient; semi-structured interviews with health professionals; participant observation and 'end of shift' handover reports. Details of these data, and the projects in which they were collected, are reported in Jones (2005) and Collins et al. (2003).

Types of nurse encounter and their different tasks

Three types of encounter are considered. One is the admission interview. This is referred to interchangeably (in nursing texts, for example, Chapman 1983: 90; and by nurses) as admission, assessment, taking a patient's history, or doing the nursing history. Its purpose is to record general information about the patient, in relation to their medical history and their activities of daily living (such as sleep patterns, dietary preferences, exercise and mobility).

A predominant feature of the interview is its question–answer format, within which the nurse takes the role of questioner. This orientation is established at the start, as illustrated in the following extract:

Extract 1 (N = nurse; P = patient)

```
N:  Righty ho (0.3) umh if it's ok with you I'll go through
    the nursing side of thing[s: with you ↑later
P:                            [alright okay ((nods))
N:  after I've asked you the quest[ions
P:                                [right
N:  and um if you want to ask me anything you'll be able to
    do so (.) al::right
P:  ye::s
```

(Audio-recorded admission interview, 342/DK)

The nurse marks the initiation of business ('righty ho'), and then proposes that they deal with 'the nursing side of things later' (line 2), after she has 'asked . . . the questions' (line 4). The patient displays his concurrence with the proposal ('alright okay ((nods))', line 3; 'yes', line 8). The nurse's proposal serves to separate other tasks (such as taking the patient's blood pressure/temperature, and making preparations for surgery), from the current task and the questions required to complete the admission and its documentation. It also creates a boundary between the nurse's questions and topical contributions from any the patient might have.

The question–answer format of these interviews is illustrated in Extract 2, from a different case. The interview proceeds through a series of standard questions asked by the nurse, who writes down the patient's answers on a form to complete the admission documentation:

Extract 2

```
N:  Do you know your weight and your height?
P:  Uh:
    (1.1)
P:  Jus' over eight stone °I am°
    (3.6) ((N is writing in the notes))
P:  and (.) five one and a half (.) °should be°
N:  Ok u::m any difficulties with your hearing or do you wear
    a hearing aid=
P:  No:
N:  No problems with hear[ing] then
P:                       [no ]
    (4.5) ((N is writing in the notes))
N:  Any visual problems::
P:  U::hm I've gorra wear glasses for reading=
N:  For reading any double vision or (.)
P:  No::
N:  No- (.) jus' glasses for reading=
P:  yeh
N:  Do you wear dentures or your [own (.) own teeth
P:                               [no
    (4.9) ((N is writing in the notes))
N:  Uh do you speak English and Welsh or jus' English
P:  English=
N:  just English
    (4.2) ((N is writing in the notes))
N:  Uhm (.) any false arms leg hip replacement knee
    replacements
```

(Audio-recorded hospital admission interview, 298/OB)

The interaction unfolds through the nurse's questions (lines 1, 7, 13, 19, 22 and 26) followed by the patient's minimal responses. Many of the answers are followed by intervals during which the nurse writes the answer in the notes (lines 5, 12, 21 and 25) before initiating her next question. The assessment progresses from questions concerning the patient's bodyweight/height, hearing, sight, through to questions relating to mobility, such as whether the patient has any false limbs. This is typical of these interviews, in which the topical remit as a whole, and the movement from one topic to a next, is generally produced in accordance with the layout and content of the form; the design of which did not lend itself to discussion or elaboration of the patient's concerns or problems.[1] Topics were generally introduced in a series according to the standard sub-headings (weight/height, sensory problems, mobility problems) printed on the assessment form.

The second type of encounter concerns the diabetes review consultation in primary care. In this consultation, the patient's latest HbA1c result, weight, current medication, lifestyle, and any prospective changes in treatment, are reviewed. These details are written into a computer template, which, like the admissions form described above, to some extent structures the interaction and its topical remit, through the nurse's questions. For example, 'you don't smoke, do you?', 'and there's no family history of heart disease or stroke, is there?', 'how much alcohol do you have in a week?', 'what about exercise?' In some instances, this nurse consultation precedes and prepares the ground for a GP consultation; in others, the nurse conducts the consultation independently. In all recorded cases, this consultation followed a series of others for the same patient, dating back over several months or years.

The third type of encounter concerns patients' consultations with the specialist cancer nurse, following their consultation with the surgeon in which a cancer diagnosis and/or options for treatment have been presented. In the specialist cancer nurse consultations, no form-filling exercise takes place. The nurse's questions do, however, govern the remit of topics to be discussed, through their orientation to points already raised by the doctor. The nurse invites the patient, through questions and prompts that reference the topics covered in the surgeon's consultation, to comment on what they have understood, and to voice their feelings and reactions to the diagnosis and to the treatment proposals or decisions. As well as exploring the topics raised during the surgeon's consultation, the nurse also raises issues relating to lifestyle, such as smoking, alcohol, and diet, and gives advice in relation to these. For each of the recordings made, this was the patient's first consultation with this nurse.

The importance of nurses' consultations with patients

These types of encounter are highly significant for a patient's care. First, in itself, the conduct of any single nurse–patient encounter has consequences for the tasks it directly addresses, for the nurse–patient relationship and for the form of their subsequent consultations. The admissions interview, for example, is often the patient's first opportunity, on arrival in hospital, to talk with a health professional. It is described by Sully and Dallas (2005: 74; see also Fitzgerald 2002: 163) as 'the foundation of all the care to follow. It is important that [the nurse] engage the others in the interview in order to develop a partnership with them.'

Second, the nurse consultation has a bearing on the patient's corresponding consultations with other health professionals. It can prepare the ground for, or consolidate talk from, the patient's other consultations. Thus it can both enhance understandings of topics talked about with the patient in those other consultations, and contribute to the maintenance of those other relationships. As one surgeon in the cancer clinic explained:

Extract 3

[The specialist cancer nurse] can't discuss the surgery probably in the same detail that I can. But she can certainly pick up on the other aspects of it in a much more humane way . . . I'm sure when I talk about speech and swallowing, it all sounds very sort of blasé and '. . . take your voice box out. Fit you with a button, you'll be right as rain' . . . Whereas she can talk about it in a much more, what it's actually like for the punter kind of approach.

(Interview with head and neck surgeon, D2-102)

A corresponding description by the specialist cancer nurse in the same clinic portrays how her consultation builds on 'what's been said', and what the patient has heard or understood, from the surgeon's consultation:

Extract 4

I tend to focus on . . . what's been said – but also 'what have you heard?' And develop it with, what were they expecting, and what did they feel . . . whether they've got 'tumour', whether they've got a 'growth', or whether the word 'cancer' has been used . . . try and explore what they've heard and what they've understood by it.

(Interview with specialist cancer nurse, A-134)

Third, patients often voice concerns to nurses that they do not tell doctors, and nurse consultations can provide distinct avenues for patients to offer their own interpretations and explanations of problems (Collins 2005a). The following account by a dietician in the cancer clinic provides one example:

Extract 5

We had a lady on the ward recently who didn't want to have surgery. She was a lady of 89 years old and needed a pharyngectomy, and she wouldn't have survived, she was a little frail old lady. And this lady

> kept telling [the specialist nurse] and I that she didn't want to have surgery, that she didn't want to have radiotherapy. But when the doctors came she told them that she did. That was really difficult and we just took the bull by the horns and [the specialist nurse] went off and said [to the doctors], 'Look, this lady doesn't want to have it.'
>
> (Interview with dietician in head and neck cancer, A-105)

Further illustration of this point is provided by comparing the topics talked about in a patient's consultations with a nurse and with a doctor, where both were recorded. A patient tended to reveal more in the nurse consultation than in the corresponding doctor one. For example, in one specialist nurse consultation, the patient said *'Another thing is, do I want to live?'* This followed immediately from a surgeon consultation in which surgery, as a possible form of treatment, had become a strong possibility. In another diabetes nurse consultation, a patient offered an explanation for the rise in his blood glucose levels – *'And with the stress of all the moving'*. In the corresponding doctor consultation, no explanations for this rise in blood glucose levels were pursued.

Forms of participation in nurse–patient encounters

Across the three types of encounter, the analyses identified certain communication features that appear to influence whether or not, and how, patients express their feelings, concerns and understandings. These features relate to the means by which the nursing tasks are realized in interaction. The analyses are presented first in relation to factors that restrict, or shape the possible form of, patients' participation, and, second, in relation to features of interaction that enhance it.

Factors that restrict (or shape the possible form of) participation

In our data, we noted two recurring factors that shape how patients participated in these encounters, and that appear to restrict their contributions. These factors pertain to how the need to accomplish particular tasks appears to make the nurse less responsive to the patients' possible contributions. To put it another way, the nurse's enactment of the task and its associated activities, such as writing on the admissions form, appear to stand in the way of the patient's expression of their concerns and understandings.

One of these factors relates to the ways in which topics are defined by the standard questions on the form or template.

In Extract 6, from an admissions interview, the nurse asks the patient how long he sleeps. The patient's initial response displays the difficulty he is having in formulating an answer to this question (line 3):

Extract 6

N: How-how long do you sleep (.) ↑for
(3.2)
P: °Uh:: I wake quite early uhm::°
N: How many hours do you sleep at night
P: Well I try and get eight hours but it's not- it's not
always eleven o'clock umh
(0.6)
N: Broken sleep ↑is it
P: I sleep till seven probably yeh yeh
(0.5)
N: How many hours a night rough::ly
(0.5)
P: Say seven um I think
(7.8) ((N writes 'sleeps seven hours a night'))
N: Righty ho you're a retired gentlema:n

(Audio-recorded hospital admission interview, 590/PD)

Through her questions, the nurse pursues a particular response – the number of hours the patient sleeps. The patient's responses (lines 3, 5–6, 9 and 13) are characterized by forms of delay, hesitation and qualification (the 3.2 second interval, line 2, that prefaces his first response; his 'uh::' in line 3; the repeat 'it's not- it's not', line 5; and the qualifiers 'well I try', line 5, 'probably', line 9). These perturbations display the difficulty the patient is having in producing an answer that fits the question. His answers convey that the amount of time he sleeps is variable ('I try and get 8 hours but . . .', line 5). In response to these difficulties, the nurse reformulates her question (lines 4 and 11). In the first reformulation, she specifies that she is looking for the number of *hours* ('how many hours do you sleep at night', line 4); and in the second reformulation, she indicates that an estimation will suffice ('how many hours a night *roughly*', line 11). In response, the patient produces an estimate ('*say* seven um *I think*', line 13), which the nurse writes down (line 14). She then proceeds to a next topic and question – the patient's employment status (line 15).

Extract 7 provides another example of the question–answer format of these admissions interviews:

Extract 7

N How much do you weigh
(1.0) ((patient turns away to think – hand to brow))
N Any idea
P Nine and a quarter I think
(2.0) ((nurse writing in the notes)
N Suffer with any disabilities or weaknesses

P No (.) no
N Arthritis or anything
P (a bit of) arthritis
(6.0) ((nurse writing in the notes)
N Does that cause you a lot of problems
P Well yeh my leg do
(12.0) ((nurse writing in the notes)
N Speaking in uh English=
P English ((laughs))
N ((laughs)) any Welsh
P No you're joking ((laughs))
N Are you in any pain or anything at the moment

(Audio-recorded hospital admission interview, 891/VE)

These examples show how the interaction is structured by the need to complete the form or template and to write down answers to the questions it dictates. Consequently, any discussion or elaboration on the topics raised is circumscribed, and the patients' contributions are minimal.

The other factor which restricts, or shapes the possible form of, patients' participation relates to the way in which, because of the presence of the task, topics and concerns that patients raise may either be met with no response by the nurse, or, where there is some discussion, are abruptly dropped in the resumption or continuation of the task. Extracts 8 and 9 provide illustration.

In Extract 8, from a diabetes review consultation, the patient raises his concern about a tablet he takes which gives him a cough (lines 1–2), and expresses his awareness of another tablet that does 'the same job' (lines 6–7):

Extract 8

P: There's two tablets, and (.) °they°gimme one type. I
(uh) get a cough.
(0.3)
N: Yeah.
(0.7)
P: And they i- bu- (0.2) I get a- (0.5) the other type I
don't. (1.0) but they both do the same ↑job.
(1.2)
N: .hhhh ↑Right Doctor ((name))'ll be waiting for you

(Video-recorded consultation in diabetes, B-114-352)

The patient relates the effects of the two types of tablets in two contrastive assessments, delivered across two turns. He first highlights the problem he has experienced with one tablet ('they gimme one type, I get a cough', lines

1–2), and follows this (after a receipting 'yeah' from the nurse, line 4) with a trouble-free evaluation of the other tablet ('. . . the other type I don't', lines 6–7). He concludes his description with a comparative 'they both do the same job'. Thus the patient provides a rationale, based on his experience of both tablets, and on his understanding that both tablets serve the same purpose, for switching from one tablet to the other. By highlighting the problem in this way, and suggesting a solution, he is making a request (albeit indirect) to alter his medication. After a 1.2-second interval, the nurse produces her next turn. In this next turn, no reference, receipt or acknowledgement of the topic of the patient's prior turns is forthcoming. The nurse's turn begins to close the consultation, with 'right', followed by an announcement of the patient's imminent appointment with the doctor ('doctor. . . . 'll be waiting for you', line 9). The patient's mention of his concern about the tablet thus closes abruptly, through reference to an impending next consultation (which the doctor is reportedly waiting to begin). The patient's concern is not followed up by the nurse in her next turn, and thus it does not achieve topical status in this consultation.

In some instances, as in Extract 9, the patient's talk is focused in a particular way, according to the nurse's agenda. This extract is from a specialist nurse consultation, in which the nurse has just asked (not shown in the transcript) the patient how he is feeling, following his consultation with the surgeon some minutes previously. The patient recounts the terror he has been feeling all morning (lines 1–2), reports his relief in response to the news delivered to him by the surgeon that his cancer is in the early stages (lines 5–6), and expresses his commitment to giving up smoking (line 10):

Extract 9

```
P:  . . . you don't know how terrified I've been all morning.
    thinking about that.=
N:  =Yeah.
    (1.0)
P:  But no::- that's smashing is that. (.)n he said it were
    in early stages. didn't he.
    (.)
N:  Yes:.
    (0.4)
P:  And I give ower smoking after this weekend.
    (0.3)
N:  °Right.° (0.3).h I'll just give you:.
    (1.3)
P:  (Matches.)
    (0.4)
N:  A little book, (.) hheh heh heh=
```

P: =Just- (.) I can't see.- (0.2) (I) can't [see
N: [NO well I- (.)
it's ALright. I'll give you this to take away. (.) which
(.) is- (.) it's just a little book about (.) stopping
smoking . . .

(Audio-recorded consultation in head and neck cancer, B-357-134)

The patient's account of the surgeon consultation is delivered over three turns, corresponding to three significant outcomes from it (relief from the terror he has been feeling, the discovery that his cancer is not as severe as it might have been, and his decision to give up smoking). In response to each, the nurse produces minimal receipt tokens ('yeah', line 3; 'yes', line 8; and 'right', line 12). In the same turn in which the nurse receipts the patient's concluding part of his account, she begins to introduce an intervention 'I'll just give you' (line 12), and, following a joky completion by the patient (line 14), proceeds to describe the intervention (line 16). The patient's mention of smoking provides the nurse with an opportunity to hand over a booklet about smoking cessation (which, as noted above, is one of the issues which she views as her responsibility to raise). In response to the nurse's completion of her introduction of this intervention, 'a little book' (line 16), the patient responds with 'I can't see . . . I can't see' (line 17). The nurse, in counter-reply, offers reassurance to the patient that he will be able to take the book away with him. This begins an extended turn in which the nurse describes how the book may be helpful in stopping smoking.

The nurse's response to the patient's account thus focuses on one part of it, the patient's expressed commitment to giving up smoking. Her response acknowledges the patient's prior turns somewhat neutrally, without responding to them topically, without evaluating or assessing them in anyway, and without any form of encouragement to the patient to continue talking. Given the patient's commitment to giving up smoking, and its congruence with the booklet she has to hand out, it is notable that the nurse does not offer more explicit acknowledgement. When the patient says he can't see well enough to read it, the nurse acknowledges this in such a way as to disregard the difficulty the patient might have in reading it ('no well it's alright', lines 18–19) – the nurse says she will give him the booklet to take away, but does not check whether he will be able to read it later. Furthermore, through the nurse's elaboration of the patient's last-mentioned topic from his consultation with the surgeon (smoking), development of topical talk on the two concerns the patient mentioned first of all (the cancer diagnosis, and his feelings of terror) is sidelined.

Communication practices that enhance patient participation

The examples presented above indicate ways in which topics are constructed and organized through the nurse's questioning, the nurse's characterizations of the task and the nurse's orientation to the agenda.

Across the set of recorded consultations, there are occasions when the interaction departs from task-oriented routines. These departures take the form of side sequences which are more conversational in character. These side sequences can be seen as having the potential to facilitate patients' involvement and to nurture the nurse–patient relationship, by allowing forms of expression and elaboration of patients' concerns that are not afforded within the constraints of completing documentation. These asides contrast with the 'formalities' of the questions on a paper form or computer template and of the procedures of admission or review.

In Extract 10, from a diabetes consultation, the nurse marks the start of business with 'right' (Walker 1994) and then introduces the task of review by reference to completion of the computer-based template (line 1):

Extract 10

```
N:  R:ight. >if we just< go through all this bit.
    (1.5)
P:  ((clears throat))
    (1.8)
P:  That's wrong.
    (1.0)
N:  What's wrong.
    (0.3)
P:  That's wrong. (0.6) hhhh[h heh heh heh=
N:                          [(Have you sh:runk). (0.3)
    =[heh heh
N:  [().
P:  .thh [hmm hah hm                [heh heh heh hah hah hah
N:       [(course you will) (.)[.hhhhh how much do you weigh
    then.
    (0.8)
P:  U::h (0.3) I don't know. (0.3) about (0.6) twenty-two I
    think, (0.6).hhhhh (0.3) maybe a bit mo:re.
```

(Audio-recorded consultation in diabetes, B-114-352)

The nurse's opening (line 1) introduces the task ('right . . .') and projects it as something to go through together ('. . . if we just go through all this bit'). Following an interval in the talk, during which the patient clears his throat (lines 2–5), the patient speaks next. In his turn, he contests the accuracy of the information portrayed on the computer template ('that's wrong'). Through this comment, the patient presents his own interpretive stance to the data displayed on the computer. The patient's comment then leads into a discussion about the patient's weight, in which the patient reveals his understanding of what his weight is, and tells the nurse that he has lost some weight *before* being weighed in this consultation.

In Extract 11, from another diabetes consultation, there is some discussion at the start of the consultation concerning the patient's sibling who has recently been diagnosed with diabetes (not shown in transcript). The nurse then marks the introduction of the business of this consultation with 'right' and proceeds with the task of review, starting with the patient's blood pressure (line 1):

Extract 11

```
N:  Right (.) if you just bob your jacket off'n we'll do yer:
    blood pressure first then.=
P:  =Right
    (1.9)
N:  Been alright yer blood pressure int? it.
    (1.2)
P:  Ye::ah since I've come down cuz av (.) I'm bin on them
    tablets a while now=
N:  =Mm.
    (4.2) ((nurse starts taking patient's blood pressure))
```

(Video-recorded consultation in diabetes, B-336-118)

As the nurse prepares to take the patient's blood pressure, she comments that it has 'been alright' (line 5). The patient agrees ('yeah'), refers to the fact that her blood pressure has come down, and links this to the tablets she has been taking, in a way which conveys their positive effect (lines 7–8). The nurse produces a minimal acknowledgement in response ('mm', line 9) and then begins to take the patient's blood pressure.

In this sequence, the patient becomes involved, through the nurse's comment (in line 5), in the production of an assessment of her blood pressure, and displays her understanding of how it has been. This sequence is an aside to the activity of taking the blood pressure; talk which arises in the preparation of this activity. As such, it provides an opportunity for comment; one in which the patient participates.

In the specialist cancer nurse consultations, the encounter is built on the surgeon's consultation it follows. In the opening, and throughout the consultation, the interaction is constructed as a series of comments arising from the surgeon's consultation that preceded it (and see Extracts 4 and 9 above). Extract 12 is from a consultation for a patient who has a throat cancer. It shows the opening of the patient's consultation with the nurse, following the surgeon consultation in which the patient received the cancer diagnosis. In that previous consultation, the surgeon had also discussed treatment, and advised that radiotherapy alone, without surgery, would be appropriate. This relieved the patient, who had reported his fear of being anaesthetized. The nurse opens the consultation by checking how the patient is feeling ('alright', line 1):

Extract 12

N: Alright.
(0.3)
P: ↑Yeah. (0.3) yeah.
(.)
N: >What do you< think to that then.
(1.4)
P: Well >I think it's a< best n.- (0.2) best un- (.) b- (.)
best option I go. >I go(t) if I'm wakened all time I'm
not bothered,
(0.3)
N: Right. (0.4) ri[ght.
P: [>You know what< I mean.
(.)
N: [Yeah.
P: [I aren't- (0.5) I'm not honestly (0.4) .hhhhhh (0.2)
>they can< take me finger off. as long as I'm wakened.

(Audio-recorded consultation in head and neck cancer, B-357-134)

In response to the nurse's initial 'alright', the patient confirms that he is feeling okay ('yeah yeah', line 3). The nurse then invites him to comment on his thoughts, in relation to what was said in that prior consultation ('what do you think to that then', line 5). The patient replies by describing the radiotherapy as 'the best option I've got', and continues by saying 'if I'm wakened all the time I'm not bothered' (lines 8–9). Thus, in this consultation, the patient has an opportunity to reflect on the treatment proposal presented to him, and to express his feelings about it. His formulation of the situation conveys his preference for radiotherapy ('the best option . . .'), and his awareness of the choice between this and surgery.

Extract 13 is from another cancer consultation, with a different patient. The extract comes in the middle of the consultation, immediately following an interruption by the surgeon, who came into the room momentarily to relay details of the pathology report that confirm the cancer diagnosis he presented to the patient in their preceding consultation. When the surgeon leaves the room, the nurse asks the patient what he understands of the diagnosis he has been given (lines 1–5):

Extract 13

N: .hh Can I just ask what you understood then (when he)
said it was a tumour. (0.8) and he's just come in and
said it confirmed what (0.7) he thought. (2.3) >well uh<
what would you- (1.2) what would you take from that. >I
mean< (1.3) in terms of what sort of tumour.
(1.9)
P: >When I say< tumours are eithe:r (0.9) benign! (0.8) or
malignant. (.) aren't they.
(.)
N: °Right°
(.)
P: If it's followed up by: (.) secondary treatment. then to
me it's malignant.
(1.0)
N: °Right.°
(3.5)
N: °(Alright).°
(0.5)
P: Otherwise he'd just whip it out and say. (.) there you
are. (0.5) that's it.
(.)
N: Sorted. (0.9) yeah

(Audio-recorded consultation in head and neck cancer, B-348-134)

In the nurse's opening turn, she invites the patient to comment on his understanding and interpretation of his situation, as it has been presented to him by the surgeon. She reports the surgeon's words 'he said it was a tumour', 'he's just come in and said it confirmed what he thought' (lines 2–3); and asks the patient 'what would you take from that', 'what sort of tumour' (lines 4–5).

In response, the patient displays his understanding that tumours are either benign or malignant (lines 7–8). He subsequently elaborates on this by demonstrating what he can infer from his own situation. The surgeon has not specified whether his tumour is benign or malignant; but the patient understands it to be malignant in his case, because, he says, it's being 'followed up by secondary treatment' (line 12), and, he continues, if it were not malignant, the surgeon would just 'whip it out and say . . . that's it' (lines 19–20).

The expression of patients' concerns, understandings and expectations

Across the three types of encounter, patients' contributions can be seen to take the form of answers that are grounded in the way in which the interview is organized and its topics prioritized through the nurse's talk. This has its influence on the possible forms that patients' participation can take.

One respect in which nurse's talk limits participation concerns the way in which topics are paced and progress through a series of questions and answers, as shown in Extracts 1, 2, 6 and 7.

A second respect in which patients' participation may be limited concerns the absences of topical follow-up, evaluation or assessment. For example, in the consultation from which Extract 6 is taken, there is no exploration of the problems with sleeping (the patient mentions waking early, and that he has no fixed bedtime) from the patient's perspective. In Extract 8, the patient raises the possibility of changing to another tablet, and one he would prefer, but this is met with no response from the nurse. In Extract 9, the patient's relief at having his cancer diagnosed as in the early stages is not responded to by the nurse.

A third form of restriction on patients' participation in the present data, related to the above, concerns the topically neutral receipts of patients' talk that the nurses produce, and the abrupt, disjunctive topic shifts they initiate. Such actions display a preoccupation with the task over the communication with the patient. They also mean that for the patient, the progression from one topic to a next may appear random. Topics may be raised without warning for the patient; and may not necessarily cover concerns the patient might have wished or chosen to raise.

A fourth restriction concerns how the routines of questions and answers are dictated by the need to complete forms and templates. The intervals during which the nurse is absorbed in writing (for example, Extract 2, line 21; Extract 6, line 14) provide the launch point for a topic switch to the next question on the assessment form. The content of the form, the size of the box to write in, the order of the questions on the computer template all influence the way in which topics are raised, characterized, progressed and closed.

As well as these restrictions and limitations on patients' participation, these data also illustrate the potential for patients to contribute. The way in which the agenda is set, and the forms of questioning and how these delimit the topical remit, may be highly routinized as the examples show, but nonetheless they offer opportunities for spontaneous talk. Thus, it seems, the constraints studied here may be lifted or turned to creative use. Particular features of the communication in these types of encounter offer potential for patients' participation. In the process of accomplishing the task, significant concerns, information, and understandings are drawn out. The asides provide outlets for conversational talk, within which the patient may make more substantive and personal contributions. For example, the joking and laughter that ensue from one patient reporting that he can only speak English, not Welsh (Extract 7); or another patient's comment that the information displayed about him on the computer screen is wrong (Extract 10).

These contributions, although minimal in most of the instances presented here, indicate something of the patient's goals, concerns and expectations. These may have little or no clinical relevance, but, without being explicated, it is not possible to know whether the patient's concerns are being addressed. As Extract 5 has illustrated, these insights into patients' understandings can be crucial, and are exactly the kind of detail that nurses are well equipped to detect, but it is a potential area of patients' participation that appears to be under-fulfilled, and compromised by the presence of various nursing tasks and roles.

Discussion: influences on participation in nurse–patient encounters

From the range of settings studied, and the examples presented in this chapter, it is clear that patients' participation in nurse consultations is shaped by a combination of influences, and cannot be explained singly in relation to factors such as time, the particular health care setting, or the task in hand. In this discussion, some of these influences are explored (see also the Educational Supplement, pp. 208–10).

First, some qualitative differences can be noted regarding the way communication proceeds in each type of encounter studied here. In the hospital admissions interviews, departures from the routine of completing the nursing assessment occur only rarely, serving to underline their institutional and highly routine character. In the diabetes review consultations, and to a lesser extent in the head and neck cancer consultations, patients already have some information and understanding from prior consultations to build on, and their actions and the ways in which they participate convey this (see Extracts 8 to 13).

Second, the examples have shown how the need to perform certain tasks of admission and review has consequences for how topics arise and are talked about, particularly in relation to the form of patients' contributions to these topics (see Extracts 1, 2, 6 and 7 above).

Third, the position and role a nurse occupies with respect to other health professionals in the team may make all the difference. With respect to the head and neck cancer setting, Extracts 3, 4 and 9 illustrate some dependence in the specialist cancer nurse consultations on topics and remits set in the preceding doctor consultation, and the subsequent effects on the characterizations of business that the nurse produces. One nurse working in diabetes who participated in our research, worked in two GP surgeries (referred to as A and B in Extract 14), and had different roles in each. In 'A', her consultations with patients were brief and confined to carrying out routine checks prior to patients' appointments with the doctor. In 'B', she ran her own diabetes clinic, with much more time for each patient. She drew the following comparison between the two types of consultation, in which she conveys not only the constraints of time, but also the influences of the doctor's respective role:

> **Extract 14**
>
> At A, it's much more task orientated and there's a doctor there and I don't really – I was certainly not involved in any of the decision-making . . . it's mainly about testing urine and taking bloods and doing blood pressure and weights . . . So there isn't really any time for any more than that. Whereas at B, the appointments are longer they're about half an hour for each patient . . . and there isn't a doctor there. I'm there on my own and a lot of the tasks are already done . . . I can actually start off by seeing where people are and just asking them about themselves and how they are and what's happening with their diabetes . . . and it's just more relaxed, more informal, and it's more possible to do diabetes education to give people information. Because you know what level they are at and they're also giving you more clues about what they need . . . I don't know what the element might be called but it's more coming from them if you like . . . rather than you sort of stamping on them what they're actually going to have done.
>
> (Interview with nurse in diabetes, A-108)

Fourth, there is the matter of the opportunities that nurse consultations provide for patients' participation. In being preparatory, or in following up, nurse's talk can offer particular kinds of opportunities for patients to contribute. In nurse consultations on which a final decision does not rest (for example, diabetes reviews which precede the patient's consultation with a doctor) nurses may be free to pursue the topics and concerns that patients present.

However, it seems that the potential of these asides for exploring patients' concerns may be understated and under-recognized. Their informality is a quality that may be lost in the bureaucracy of forms (the lack of space, the need to move to the next question), and in the organization of care. The nurse's orientation to the task may mean that patients' concerns are minimized. And while patients' concerns may often first arise in nurse consultations, nurses are not always sufficiently in the know to be able to advise patients fully, or illuminate their understanding. In situations where information isn't passed from nurse to doctor, patients' concerns and treatment preferences may be left unaddressed. These nurse consultations demonstrate the capacity for patients to contribute and to display what they are thinking. Discussions in nurses' consultations may often be extensive and elaborate, when complementing doctors' consultations and preparing (or consolidating) the topical ground of those other consultations by highlighting problems and their details. However, in being encumbered with certain tasks, limits are placed on the extent to which, in the nurse consultation, the problem can be talked about and on the import accorded to it. In these respects, the greater involvement that nursing envisages (as discussed in the introduction to this chapter) can turn out to be much more limited.

In seeking to understand patients' participation and in considering how to enhance the potential of patients' participation in their consultations with nurses, we propose that at least the following three areas be addressed. First, patients interact with teams, and by taking an interdisciplinary view of patients' participation, this dimension is accommodated. Single consultations only provide part of the picture; and the challenge of involving patients and providing opportunities for them to take an active part in their care, if they so wish, is one that demands the concerted effort of all health professionals involved, across a series of consultations.

Second, questions concerning patient participation need to be considered both in the details of instances of interaction and in relation to their broader context; that is, with reference to team-working, policy expectations, the importance of nurses' relationships with patients, and their contact time.

Third, the kinds of guidance that nurses are given in how to communicate with patients and how to provide opportunities for their participation can, we believe, be informed by understandings of the interactional dynamics of, and the contextual influences on, nurse–patient encounters. For example, the tension between performing nursing tasks and being patient-centred and according priority to communication is something that textbooks do not currently address. On the basis of the findings presented here, guidance could be given as to how to integrate the performance of a nursing task with communication and with the patient's involvement. To give another example, the details and nuances of how patients' concerns arise in their consultations with nurses would provide a useful addition to the current and widespread recommendations that patients' concerns must be addressed (which are not generally accompanied by descriptions of how to do this). Furthermore, in any encounter, the particular constraints that govern how patients are involved and the extent of their influence on interaction are likely to shift from one moment to a next. Making this point clear, in guidelines for communicating with patients, would highlight the potential for patients' involvement and participation in any nurse–patient encounter, regardless of the presence of other tasks, the constraints of time, and so on.

These angles on patient participation pose challenges for practice, for education, and for the design of research in health care communication. A broader collaborative vision is needed (Williams 2000); one which is reflected in research design, in practice across a variety of settings, in the setting of expectations and standards in policy documents, in textbooks, and in acknowledgements of how tasks are enacted through communication, in any health care encounter.

Conclusion

The types of nurse–patient encounter studied here have shown ways in which nurses' talk constrains opportunities presented for patients to contribute. They also illustrate the kinds of informal opportunities that nurses' talk presents for patients' concerns to be raised, not only for that consultation, but also for reviewing, or rehearsing, talk which takes place in other consultations. This is a potential which could be exploited to enhance patients' participation in their care.

Note

1. The initial assessment form consists of a grid of 12 squares. Each square is allocated one 'activity of living' (based on Roper et al.'s (1996) initial nursing assessment tool) to be assessed, such as sleep, mobility, diet and elimination. The squares measure approximately 6 × 4 cm. Nurses usually read the form from left to right and top to bottom, and the introduction of each topic appears random, as the form presents no logical sequencing to the areas to be assessed.

Recommendations: summary

- Set the scene at the beginning so as to maximize opportunities for the patient's contributions while carrying out necessary tasks. For example, 'This is an admissions interview. Its purpose is *x*, but it is also an opportunity for you to tell me *y*.' Or, 'In your consultation with the doctor, *x* was covered. The purpose of this one is *y*. What do you think we should discuss?'
- Employ comments on, and asides to, the task to explore patients' concerns and understandings. Expressions of sympathy or empathy, such as 'I'm sorry you don't sleep well', may provide an opening for the patient to elaborate.
- Review team dynamics. For example, it may be possible to make more explicit links between different professionals' consultations, and to share information about recurrent topics or individual patients' care.
- Consider how the available time might be organized differently to increase the chance for patients to raise issues, for example, by rearranging the topics on the assessment form to suit the individual patient.

PART III

A Conceptual Overview of Patient Participation and its Components

9 Components of participation in health care consultations

A conceptual model for research

Anssi Peräkylä and Johanna Ruusuvuori

Commentary

In this chapter and Chapter 10, the contributions to this book are presented in two conceptual overviews of patient participation. The first of these, presented here, is a model for research.

In this model for research, five components of patient participation have been identified by drawing upon the studies in this book. These are: (1) the patient's contribution to direction of action; (2) the patient's influence in the definition of the agenda of the consultation; (3) the patient's share in the reasoning processes; (4) the patient's influence in decision-making; and (5) emotional reciprocity. When taken together, these components provide a model for researching patient participation at a micro-level. Each of the five components requires specific research methods for its investigation.

This model provides a means of reviewing the research results and methods used in the studies in this book, and reflecting on their particular strengths and weaknesses. It can also be used for the planning and conduct of future research on the topic. In the discussion, applications of this model in research and practice in the field of patient participation are explored, and gaps to be filled in future research are highlighted.

Introduction

In this brief reflection upon the empirical chapters of this book, we will outline five key components of patient participation in health care consultations. 'Patient participation' is, as the studies in this book have shown, a rather multi-faceted phenomenon. In this chapter, we will break down this phenomenon into its components. The way that we break it down arises directly from the observations reported in the earlier chapters of this book. In describing the key components of patient participation, we refer to each of the earlier chapters, with a special focus on the patient's point of view.

Five key components of patient participation

We suggest that there are five key components of patient participation. The five components comprise: (1) the patient's *contribution to the direction of action*; (2) the patient's *influence in the definition of the consultation's agenda*; (3) the patient's *share in the reasoning process*; (4) the patient's *influence in the decision-making*; and (5) the *emotional reciprocity* between the patient and the provider of the care. These components, sites and methods are illustrated in Table 9.1. Following this, we will detail each component in turn, drawing on examples from the previous chapters. In relation to each component, we will show its specific site of empirical manifestation, and we will also show

Table 9.1 Five key components of patient participation

Component	*Site of empirical manifestation*	*Research method*
1. Patient's contribution to the direction of action, for example: – question–answer sequences – delivery and reception of diagnosis – delivery and reception of treatment recommendations	The sequence – initiatory acts – responsive acts The turn	CA Think aloud interviews
2. Patient's influence in the definition of the consultation's agenda	Consultation Sequence	CA Think aloud interviews
3. Patient's share in the reasoning process	Sequence Consultation	Interviews Think aloud CA
4. Patient's influence in the decision-making	Sequence Consultation Patient journey	Interviews Focus groups CA
5. Emotional reciprocity	Sequence Consultation .Patient journey	Interviews CA

how, to be properly understood, each component requires specific research methods.

The patient's contribution to the direction of action

The patient's contribution to the direction of action involves the ways in which the patient takes the initiative in shaping the action sequences of which the consultation consists. Action sequences include, for example, the delivery and reception of the reason for consultation, question–answer sequences in professional–patient (or researcher–patient) interviews, the delivery and the reception of diagnosis, and the delivery and the reception of treatment recommendations.

The patient's contribution to action sequences can occur in two positions: as an *initiation* or as a *response*. When the patient initiates an action sequence, they put the professional in a position where the professional is expected to respond to the patient's initiation. The patient can take the initiative, for example, by asking a question or by asking for advice. The delivery of the presenting problem can also be considered as such an initiation. In very general terms, we can propose that the more opportunities the patient has for initiatory actions, the more the patient participates in directing a consultation. Although patients' initiatory actions do not receive much attention in the chapters of this book, there are some references to them. In Extract 1 of Chapter 6 (Gafaranga and Britten), for example, the patient takes the initiative in asking whether they have to keep taking their pills. Gafaranga and Britten indicate that the patient's question serves the purpose of showing the patient's negative stance towards medication. A very similar example, in which the patient raises their preference for taking a different tablet from the one they are currently prescribed, is Extract 8 of Chapter 8 (Jones and Collins). Patients' initiatory actions as sites of participation is clearly one area that needs to be examined in the future (see also Drew 2001, and the exercises for this chapter).

As researched in this book, many of the patient's contributions to the direction of action involve *responses* to the professional's acts. The patient responses include, most notably, answers to questions, and responses to treatment recommendations and diagnoses. Even though the patient is in a responsive position when performing all these actions, the strength of their response may vary. This variation is crucial in developing a nuanced understanding of patient participation. The patient can, for example, give a minimal answer to the question or expand the answer in their own initiative (Stivers and Heritage 2001). An expansion of the patient's answer is shown in Extract 8 in Chapter 5 (Chatwin et al.) where the patient first answers the doctor's question regarding what he would like to be called, and then, having answered, the patient continues jokingly by referring to the various names his wife has for him. This expansion of the patient's answer may be seen as an indication of the development of a rapport between the doctor and the patient, but also as an initiative by the patient to verify and bring out in the open the more relaxed interactional dynamic that has been created. Likewise, in responding to a diagnosis or a treatment decision, the patient can merely acknowledge the doctor's proposal or can produce an extended response that displays his or her stance to the proposal. Chapter 7 (Peräkylä et al.) shows how patients take up the opportunity to participate in diagnostic discussion in response to the doctor's diagnostic statement. We also saw how patients were able to participate in the homoeopathic treatment discussion in a similar sequential place. In psychoanalytic sessions it seemed that the patients' rather elaborate responses to analysts' interpretations were constitutive of the actual task of these encounters, thus, patient participation was essential in terms of the purpose of the whole encounter. Patients' responses were also an integral part of the analyses in Chapters 6 and 8. For example, in Chapter 6, the patients' contributions were seen to shape the definition of the consultation as a follow-up or a new consultation in giving their first concerns as a response to doctors' elicitors.

To be understood through research, each component of participation requires a particular method or methods. The first component, the patient's contribution to the direction of action, requires a method that focuses on the design and organization of utterances, because it is at this micro-level of interaction where the choices regarding the direction of action are made. Conversation analysis (hereafter CA) is a method particularly apt for the investigation of these issues (and see Chapter 1). However, interviews and think aloud techniques can also be helpful, particularly, perhaps, when combined with CA. Examples of their beneficial combination are offered in Chapter 2 (Bugge and Jones).

The patient's influence on the definition of the consultation's agenda

The patient's influence on the definition of the consultation's agenda is the second component of participation. Health care consultations are typically organized around a problem or problems that need to be solved or dealt with, both in first visits and follow-up visits. The patient's influence, in defining the problem or problems to be dealt with, varies. In first visits, the key question is the patient's success in conveying their concern or concerns: in particular, the delivery of 'additional concerns' may be difficult. In follow-up visits, the patient may have concerns other than the initial reason for the follow-up, and again, they may be more or less successful in having them included in the agenda. Chapter 4 (Stevenson) brings to the fore the importance that patients place on doctors listening to their agendas. One indication of patients' influence on the agenda is given in Chapter 6, Extract 2, where the patient reminds the doctor of the purpose of the consultation and the doctor corrects his own wrong assumption as a result. In Chapter 8 (Jones and Collins), on the other hand, some examples show that people may not succeed in participating in the definition of the agenda even though they might like to.

In exploring the patients' chances for influencing the consultation agenda, one central issue is the professionals' obligation to orient to tasks other than those that arise directly from the patients' concerns. For instance, Chapter 8 shows how nurses' concentration on their institutional task, and the structuring of the encounter according to various organizational or bureaucratic constraints (such as forms to be completed) may result in patients' concerns being unexplored or undocumented. Chapter 8 also shows how departures from the routinized question–answer format may give rise to more informal types of interaction which can help to maintain the nurse–patient relationship and which thus enhance patients' influence on the construction of the agenda.

The research methods capable of investigating this component of participation are interviews, think aloud techniques and conversation analysis. Through interviews and think aloud techniques, it is possible to explore, for example, what the patient's concerns were before seeing the professional, the patients' understandings of the ways in which they had the opportunity to air these concerns during the consultation, and the ways in which these concerns were taken up by the professional. Conversation analysis may be helpful, both on its own and along with interviews, as means of investigating in detail the opportunities and obstacles, in the structure of the interaction, relating to the delivery and uptake of the patient's concerns.

The patient's share in the reasoning process

While the second component focuses on patients' influence on the topic of the consultation, the third component, *the patient's share in the reasoning process*, concentrates on the ways in which, and the extent to which, patients have a role in discussing the origins of, and potential solutions to, the problem that has been raised. On the one hand, this component concerns the patient's opportunities to convey their relevant knowledge regarding the ailment to the professional: through the description of symptoms and in the expression of the patient's understandings regarding the illness. On the other hand, this component of participation concerns the flow of information in the reverse direction: how the doctor informs the patient about the diagnosis, prognosis, and treatment. Finally, the patient's share in the reasoning process concerns the diagnostic reasoning itself: whether or not the patient has access to, and takes part in making, the inferences from symptoms to diagnosis or from symptoms to treatment decision.

In Chapter 7 (Peräkylä et al.), we saw how the professionals could give more or less room for the patient to comment upon their diagnostic or treatment suggestions. Thus, again, CA can give us information about the practices that facilitate or block participation within sequences of adjacent actions by health professionals and patients. As for the other research methods, interviews and think aloud protocols are particularly powerful here. Interviews can indicate what patients report themselves to have understood of the practitioner's way of thinking, or how patients evaluate the possibilities for their participation in the reasoning process. Various examples of this can be found in Chapter 4 (Stevenson). Think aloud protocols can expose the professional's and the patient's reasoning processes, with their possible divergences and convergences, during the course of the consultation. An example of the way in which an occasion of think aloud exposed a patient's method of reasoning that could not be located with CA, is found in Extract 3 in Chapter 2 (Bugge and Jones).

The patient's influence on the decision-making

The fourth component of participation involves *the patient's influence on the decision-making*. Decisions concerning treatment or concerning further medical investigations are the major output of the consultation process, so this component links back to all prior ones. The patient can influence these decisions and outputs in varying degrees, by proposing treatments or tests, and by taking a particular stance in relation to the doctor's proposals. This latter aspect is illuminated especially in Chapter 7, in which the possibilities for patients to participate, as offered through the ways in which the professionals design their proposals, are described. We might consider that as well as professionals providing better opportunities for participation in decision-making through the ways in which they present information about their decisions, they could also provide several options for the patient to choose from, instead of presenting only one.

A different way to look at patients' influence on decision-making is to explore their views and preferences with regard to participation in decision-making. Interviewing and focus groups are two appropriate research methods for this. Chapter 3 (Thompson), for instance, shows that, from the patients' point of view, participation is not always even desirable. In that study, patients' preferences for involvement were found to vary on a scale, from no desire to participate at one end, to an interest in autonomous decision-making at the other. Similar differences were observed in Chapter 4 (Stevenson). While the data presented in that chapter showed how patients generally favoured consultations that enabled participation, there were also patients who spoke for more passive models pointing out the responsibility of the professional.

Emotional reciprocity

Emotional reciprocity is the fifth component of patient participation. This component concerns the patient's opportunities for the expression of emotions during the consultation, and health professionals' responses to these displays, as well as patients' experiences of consultations and of health professionals' behaviour. At the micro-interactional level, emotion displays take place through the design of utterances and the relations between them. An example of this is offered in Chapter 8 (Jones and Collins), illustrating how departures from the routinized question–answer format may bring opportunities for more informal types of interaction that can help to maintain the nurse–patient relationship. Chapter 5 (Chatwin et al.) shows how emotional reciprocity is built as the professional works to undo the conventional expectations towards a medical consultation with various techniques, such as discussing the patient's willingness to be video-taped, and sounding out the patient's preference as to how he would like to be addressed. This chapter also shows how the homeopath gradually unravels the patient's expectations that may have developed during their previous encounters with conventional health care. Likewise, the importance of emotional reciprocity was documented in Chapter 4 (Stevenson), where patients' views on 'good' and 'bad' consultations were analysed. From the interviews presented in that chapter, it became clear that the patients valued doctors who were considerate, understanding and interested, and that doctors who listened were also felt to encourage patient participation.

Emotional reciprocity can thus be investigated through CA, which can expose features of the interactional organization of emotion, as well as through interviews and focus groups, which can offer access to what the patients or the professionals did *not* reveal in their actual face-to-face encounter.

Discussion

In sum, the five components of patient participation outlined above constitute a conceptual model for reflecting upon, planning and conducting research in this field (and see the Educational Supplement, pp. 210–12). The model serves to illuminate the strengths and weaknesses of specific research methods in analysing a particular manifestation of patient participation. In more general terms, CA (like other observational methods) is an apt method for analysing participants' actions and procedures taken *during* the actual consultation *process* (see Chapters 5, 6, 7 and 8). With a conversation analysis based on recorded data, it is possible to pinpoint procedures that enhance or weaken patient participation in the consultation. The method makes possible a detailed description of ongoing interaction, and of specific actions taken with their specific consequences. Another method that can be used to analyse the actual process of medical consultation (see Chapter 8) is non-participant observation. Unlike CA, this method does not produce replayable data and thus does not allow for the checking of the analytic interpretations made. It therefore usually needs other methods, such as interviews, to support it. However, it may be particularly useful in situations where recording is difficult or impossible (e.g. when a patient moves from one location to another during their visit to hospital). While CA and non-participant observation give information on the process of medical consultation, there is much they do not tell us. They do not (directly) tell us about what goes on in people's minds, about their subjective explanations for choosing specific ways of acting among a range of possibilities, about how people experience their possibilities to participate, or about their views on participation in general. Retrospective think aloud (Chapter 2) and interviews and focus groups (Chapters 3, 4, 5 and 8) are methods that provide this sort of information. Interviews may be conducted one-to-one, between the researcher and one interviewee (Chapter 4), but also in focus groups (Chapter 3) and themed discussions (Chapter 5) where instead of just asking questions the researcher acts as moderator in a discussion between various individuals and/or representatives of particular interest groups. Interviews and focus groups provide information on people's opinions and experiences outside the actual consultation. However, one must remember that they are not necessarily any more accurate in describing what people actually think or feel than CA or non-participant observation. Instead, they give an outlook on what interviewees decide to tell interviewers in a research interview. In contradistinction to the observational methods of CA, the interview situation is initiated by the researcher for research purposes, and thus has particular objectives with distinct roles for each participant which guide them in their conversation.

Further, as was suggested in Chapter 2, it may sometimes be beneficial to combine several methods in order to analyse a particular phenomenon. In such cases, however, it is important to remember that different methods afford different views on the phenomenon studied, and that, because of this, the research questions that can be posed using a specific method must also be different. Different methods provide different types of information about the same subject of research, and this should be taken into account when thinking about combining methods in one study.

This model of the components of participation presents a summary of the research results presented, and of the methods used, in the chapters of this book. Thus, it also helps to point out potential gaps in present approaches to patient participation. One obvious gap is the lack of research on the patients' initiatory acts. This deficiency has also been identified by others, for example, Drew (2001: 263) pointed out that patients' objectives may be 'manifest in the interactional initiatives that patients make'. This is one area in which more research is clearly needed. A further absence concerns the fact that most of the chapters in this book deal with physician–patient encounters. In Chapter 7 (Peräkylä et al.), we saw how we can find both similarities and differences in analysing a similar action in three different types of medical consultations. Chapter 5 (Chatwin et al.) points to some distinctive qualities of homoeopathic consultations, and Chapter 8 (Jones and Collins) refers, albeit indirectly, to some differences between nurses' and doctors' communication. Such comparisons would be beneficial in both locating potential practices that enhance patient participation, as well as in gaining knowledge about the particular qualities of different types of consultations and their equivalent participant roles. Finally, one further 'omission' of this book is its exclusive focus on qualitative studies. It might be considered that, ideally, the model of components that these studies have made available could also inform further quantitative studies on patient participation.

Recommendations: summary

- In planning research on patient participation, it is important to consider the method with regard to the phenomenon to be studied. Thus, for example, CA is well-suited to the study of patients' participation during the actual consultation process, whereas interviews and focus groups provide information on people's opinions and experiences outside the actual consultation.
- It may sometimes be beneficial to combine several methods in order to analyse a particular phenomenon. In such a case, however, caution should be exercised when summing up the results and making generalizations: different methods provide different types of information on the same subject of research. This means that the individual results of two different methods may not strictly represent the same phenomenon.

10 An integrative approach to patient participation in consultations

Andrew Thompson, Johanna Ruusuvuori, Nicky Britten and Sarah Collins

Commentary

In this final and concluding chapter, we return to questions originally posed in Chapter 1, to review the distinct contributions and insights afforded by the research on patient participation presented in this book. These questions are: What is participation? Can we recommend it? Can we measure it?

In providing some answers to these questions, we employ a conceptual framework to integrate the ideas and themes of the book. This framework is intended to reflect the multi-faceted nature of patient participation, which, we suggest, can be understood in terms of components, levels and contexts. Within this framework, we suggest that distinctions should be made between desired and achieved levels of participation; and that, because not all patients want to participate at all times, participation cannot be understood in global terms but only in specific settings and types of consultations.

This framework is intended to facilitate identification of the linkages and contributions that can be made, across different research approaches and disciplines, in the study of patient participation. It also enables identification of gaps that potentially need to be filled. It aims to demonstrate how these various studies may enable patients and their organizations, health care practitioners, managers and policy-makers to advance their understanding of this taken-for-granted, yet opaque, concept that is high on the policy agenda.

Finally, we identify and discuss possible avenues for future research.

Introduction

We have emphasized the need for an integrated approach to the study of patient participation throughout this book. In Chapter 1, we outlined some previously developed constituents of patient participation. In Chapter 2 we summarized the use of multiple approaches in studying patient participation, to outline the breadth and depth of the contributions in this book, and to invite explorations between methods and perspectives. Chapters 3–8 made reference to consultation recordings and to the expressed views of patients and health professionals, in order to elucidate particular features of patient participation. In following on from the findings presented in those chapters, Chapter 9 developed a conceptualization of the key components of patient participation, to foster more detailed and empirically grounded research on the topic. This final chapter continues the book's interdisciplinary theme, by integrating the substantive threads into a holistic framework for the study and practice of patient participation.

This framework has three aims. The first is to map the findings of the various studies contained in the book, to show how they contribute to a more comprehensive and sophisticated analysis of the concept of patient participation than has hitherto been available. The second aim of this framework is to provide a means by which health professionals, patient representatives, researchers and others can locate their particular practice, experience, or research in relation to patient participation. The third aim is briefly to identify gaps in understanding that need to be addressed in order to enhance knowledge and understanding of this field.

Through the presentation of this framework, we consider a number of questions that were first raised in Chapter 1.

What is patient participation?

The studies represented in this book convey the diversity of definitions of the concept of patient participation. Rather than trying to achieve a uniform view of what participation is, this book has brought these definitions into dialogue with each other.

The broadest view of patient participation, stated explicitly in Chapter 7 and echoed elsewhere, is that it is not possible to avoid participating in a consultation. Bodily presence, looking, talking, and even the acts of silence and refraining from talking, it is argued, have their influence on what happens next in a consultation. Thus any action, or withholding of action, can be said to exhibit participation.

Participation can be seen to be dependent on the contributions of all parties concerned. In many of the consultation activities studied in this book, this participation is made evident through spoken actions (for example, the formulations presented in Chapter 6). Other cases also illustrate ways in which patients may refrain from contributing verbally (see Chapter 2, Extract 2) and point to ways in which other non-verbal activities (such as writing in the patient's notes, Chapter 8) shape the possible forms of participation.

Participation may also be expressed from another angle: that is, in terms of people's views about their involvement in consultations. When asked to explain their understanding of their role in their consultations (see Chapter 3), patients and members of the public may confine participation to a particular part of the spectrum of involvement possibilities. Their accounts of what participation means, given outside the consultation, tend to be based on expectations of reciprocal relations of openness, mutual respect and the sharing of information that lead to dialogue. These qualities are echoed in the views of patients presented in Chapter 4. At the other end of this spectrum of reported involvement, there are those who would rather opt out of what they view to be any kind of involvement, by confining themselves to answering questions from the practitioner or relying on significant others to act on their behalf. Various reasons are given for preferring to opt out, including a high level of trust in the health professional, or because involvement brings responsibilities.

As found in previous studies, those patients who contributed their views in Chapter 4 stressed the importance of professionals being able to gauge the appropriate levels of involvement for individual patients and their situations. The key to this lies in being able to individualize the care provided, by tailoring information to patients' needs and understanding. Some patients said that they welcomed opportunities for participation as offering the possibility of feeling understood and being reassured, being treated respectfully and as equals. Professional knowledge and technical skills alone are not viewed as positively; and this underlines the importance of communication.

Other dimensions of patient participation are revealed by comparing the different types of health care encounter and consultation activity studied in this book, with respect to Chapters 5, 6, 7 and 8.

One dimension, also illustrated in the views of patients outlined above, concerns qualities such as rapport, empathy and openness in the health care consultation. Chapter 5 demonstrates the part these play in the opening of a therapeutic consultation in a homoeopathic hospital, and the active contributions that the patient makes to the development of these qualities; and compares this to the opening of a consultation in clinical genetics in which such qualities are not evident. Similar qualities of rapport and openness are highlighted through a nurse's description of her contrasting experience of working in different roles in different settings (Extract 14, Chapter 8).

Another dimension concerns the specific health care context. As shown in Chapter 5, consultations that integrate allopathic and complementary medicine, because of the principles on which they are based, foster feelings of equality and rapport that may not be present to the same degree elsewhere. In the psychoanalytic consultations described in Chapter 7, patient participation appears particularly salient. The interpretative sequence is treated as incomplete by the psychoanalyst if the patient does not verbally contribute. Thus, with respect to this activity and this type of consultation, these patients' contributions are accentuated beyond those found in the other consultations and activities (such as diagnosis in general practice, treatment proposals in homoeopathy) with which they are compared.

Another dimension concerns what happens in particular consultation phases and activities. Take, for example, the presentation of treatment options in consultations. In relation to this activity, patients appear to be placed in a responsive mode, regardless of the type of consultation (see Chapters 2, 5 and 7). As described in Chapter 7, patients' participation in homoeopathic treatment decisions may have more to do with working towards acceptance of the homoeopathic practitioner's proposal, than with the patient's participation in the actual decision.

A further dimension concerns the organizational agenda of the health professional. Some of the nurse–patient consultations presented in Chapter 8 demonstrate the need for nurses to fulfil certain task requirements, particularly in the case of hospital admissions interviews. The nurses' management of the consultation overall, and the series of questions put to the patient, reflect this task orientation.

Particular health professional groups, as well as types of consultation, may engender patient participation. The opening of the consultation in a homoeopathic hospital presented in Chapter 5, and the accompanying material from a themed discussion involving a GP and a homoeopath, suggest that there may be enhanced opportunities for patients' participation in consultations which are designedly holistic in approach. In Chapter 8, some qualities of nurses' consultations with patients are outlined that suggest that patients may divulge more of their concerns to nurses than they do to doctors.

These insights into the meaning of patient participation demonstrate the multiple forms that patient participation can take. They illustrate the need to attend both to what people say about how patients participate, and how patients actually participate, in their interactions with health professionals. They show that, in the context of different consultation activities, patient participation may take particular forms. Overall, they highlight the importance – for health professionals, patient organizations, policy-makers and researchers – of attending to different facets of patient participation, in order to develop a more comprehensive and nuanced understanding of the concept.

In an attempt to comprehend the multiple forms and levels of patient involvement and participation, the holistic framework presented in this chapter comprises three elements: components, levels and contexts. By approaching the concept of patient participation in terms of this framework, highly specified aspects of the consultation can be focused on. This degree of specification is important for a number of reasons. First, it engenders increased sensitivity to the various dimensions and forms that patient participation can take. Second, it invites consideration of the variability that exists at the micro-level and of the interactional dynamics of a consultation. Third, it enables a view of patient participation that is multi-faceted and that, in relation to any individual patient's experience, recognizes the interplay of a number of dimensions. Fourth, and following on from the above, it guards against making premature generalizations about the consultation as a whole. Finally, it accommodates the changing and multiple forms of patient participation in their interactive environment, in recognition of the fact that patient participation has to be seen as a continuing project.

Components of patient participation

This element, already discussed in Chapter 9, itemizes five key components of patient participation in health care encounters. Each chapter deals with one or more of these components. For the purpose of understanding what patient participation is and how it works in a consultation, it is important to note that participation can vary with respect to each of these components within the same encounter. For example, in relation to 'the patient's influence in definition of the consultation's agenda', an individual patient may wish to have the opportunity to present their interpretation of what the problem might be, to inform the diagnosis; while, in relation to 'the patient's influence in the decision-making', the same patient may prefer the health professional to take the lead. The ways in which participation varies relates to what Peräkylä and Ruusuvuori (Chapter 9) describe as empirical sites of manifestation of these components: namely, the design of individual turns and sequences of talk; the consultation as a whole; and the patient's journey. The 'emotional reciprocity' component, for example, can steadily build across one, and across multiple, consultations in a patient's journey, as in homoeopathic or general practice encounters, or as in a patient's series of visits to the nurse for review of their diabetes.

Levels of patient participation

The second element of the framework concerns 'levels' of patient participation. These levels concern the intended or desired degree of involvement by patients, as reported in Chapter 3. These levels are 'non-involvement', 'information-seeking/information-receptive', 'information-giving/dialogue', 'shared decision-making', and 'autonomous decision-making'.

The chapters that explored patient participation in relation to the interactional dynamics of consultations, drawing on actual recorded instances, did not specifically relate their findings to these levels. However, by reflecting on their findings, it is possible to make links between details of the interaction, and the accounts given in Chapters 3 and 4, to evidence these levels of patient participation. In general, the examples given in this book illustrate instances of patient–professional interaction and professional activity in relation to the level of 'information-seeking/information-receptive'. In terms of health professionals' orientations to the five levels, Chapter 7 describes some differences between the various types of medical practice, with greater emphasis on the level of 'information-giving/dialogue' in the fields of homoeopathy and psychoanalysis than in general practice. A closer look at the distinct features of these different types of medical practice reveals a more dialogical approach in the development of interpretations in psychoanalysis consultations: as Peräkylä et al. put it (Chapter 7), the patient's response 'can be part of a dialogical process where the participants collaboratively construct a verbal description of the patient's mind'. By drawing comparisons across the different health care settings and types of encounter represented in this book, it is possible to consider the potential for a communication practice found in one setting to translate into others, in order to promote patients' participation.

Another aspect of these levels of patient participation concerns the potential for patients to move from one level to another. This potential relates in part to the interactional processes of consultations; and to what has been described in Chapter 9 as the position of the patient's contribution to the direction of action in a consultation. The studies in this book have been primarily concerned with sequences and activities in which the patient's contribution is responsive to, and follows from, the health professional's contribution. However, some situations have also been explored in which these positions are reversed, with, for example, the patient (or their lay carer) taking the initiative in either seeking or giving information to the professional (see, for example, Extracts 8 and 10, Chapter 8). Chapter 3 reveals that for some patients in some circumstances this is their desired position; but it is one that the professional can block. Some of the data illustrate the potential for professionals to engineer situations where patients can be put in first position, from which point the patient may take the initiative, or make the final decision (for example, line 16, Extract 8, Chapter 5).

Contexts of patient participation

The third element of the holistic framework for patient participation concerns contextual influences. Within this element, a number of different structural conditions contribute to the forms and dimensions of patient participation. The structural conditions considered here are the nature of the health problem, and the organizational setting of the encounter. Alongside these structural conditions, the role of human agency needs to be taken into account. Human agency is the ability of willing individuals and collectives to make a difference to the social systems of which they are part, in distinction to the social structures, institutions and norms that mould their field of action. Together, structure and agency help to determine the interactive space of the consultation.

In relation to the structural conditions that are imposed by the nature of the health problem, one distinction concerns whether the problem is chronic or acute; and whether the problem requires continuity of care or urgency of response. Patients with both acute and chronic health problems were specifically sampled in Chapter 3, and they accordingly revealed less or more willingness to be involved. For example, some patients with chronic illnesses, such as diabetes or asthma, expressed support for autonomous decision-making. Reflecting on his recent experiences of consultations with his GP, one patient with diabetes commented on how, if he were the doctor, he would be encouraging patients to become more autonomous and to take greater control of their illness (Extract C, educational supplement to Chapter 2, p. 202). By contrast, some patients with acute problems and relatively little medical knowledge of their problem manifested a reluctance to become involved at any level. The continuity of care dimension influences, for example, the design of the health professional's 'first concern elicitors' in the opening sequence of the consultation (Chapter 6); as well as the way in which patients consult one health professional and then another, in the review of a chronic illness such as diabetes (see Chapter 8). In terms of urgency, a number of examples in this book have shown how increased severity of illness might reduce willingness to become involved in a consultation. In such situations, patients and their carers may express a desire to trust professionals as a way of coping with fear and anxiety, or to avoid the possibility of knowing too much about a treatment and consequently losing faith in it. Chapter 3 also indicates that involvement might be more problematic for those patients who might be in need of emergency care rather than more routine forms of health care, as well as for people suffering from psychological distress, or with poor cognitive ability.

The other set of structural variables considered in this book relates to the organisational frameworks within which these health conditions are diagnosed and treated. The consultations studied in this book are mainly those between patients and GPs (referenced in Chapters 3, 4, 5, 6 and 7). The other consultations that are studied involve nurses in primary care and in hospital inpatient and outpatient settings (Chapter 8), homoeopaths (Chapters 5 and 7) and psychoanalysts (Chapter 7), and reference is also made to clinical genetics (Chapter 5), family planning (Chapter 2), and surgeon consultations in head and neck cancer (see the educational supplements to Chapters 5 and 9). These distinctive professional cultures are placed within specific organizational settings. In these examples there is a clear emphasis on the activity, time and role constraints under which allopathic medicine and nursing, whether in hospitals or in primary care environments, are seen to operate. In Chapter 8, for example, nursing is shown to be a profession that is imbued with a large bureaucratic responsibility for following protocols, completing paperwork, and generally working to support the tasks of the medical professional. Chapter 5, in the presentation of extracts from a themed discussion between a GP and homoeopath, illustrates the different organizational and environmental influences on their respective consultations.

The counterpart to the structural conditions that influence patients' participation in health care consultations is human agency, which shows itself in the positions patients and professionals choose to take, through their own strategies and actions. From the contributions to this book, three variables relating to human agency can be isolated. These variables are professionals' roles, patients' roles, and patient trust in the health professional.

Health professionals' roles

In considering health professionals' roles, four influences have been taken into account: (1) professional stocks of interactional knowledge (SIKs) that inform professionals' approaches to their consultations; (2) particular aspects of professionals' communication toolkits; (3) the role of individual professionals within teams; and (4) professionals' attitudes.

In relation to the first of these, professional stocks of interactional knowledge, Peräkylä et al. (Chapter 7) contrast the SIKs of the three types of health professional (GP, homoeopath and psychoanalyst) to show how they variously engage with patients to fulfil their strategic goals. Gafaranga and Britten (Chapter 6) show how GPs' deployment of action formulation reveals an underlying project, namely, to secure the patient's expressed commitment to doing what the GP recommends, even when there has not been any agreement. The second area of influence, that is the professionals' toolkit for interaction, includes, among other elements, the qualities of empathy, naturalness and mutuality in therapeutic consultations in Chapters 5 and 7; similar characteristics of 'good' consultations presented in Chapter 4 (such as Extract 7); and the informal talk that arises in nurses' consultations with patients (Chapter 8) and on which doctors reportedly depend to complement their own consultations (see Extract 3, Chapter 8). A third area of influence on professional roles discussed in Chapter 8 concerns the relative positions and contributions of different health professionals within a team. The fourth area of influence, health professionals' attitudes, is given explicit attention in patients' evaluations of their consultations, as presented in Chapter 4. Stevenson shows how GPs' behaviour, such as being abrupt or patronizing, can provoke negative feelings among patients. These behaviours might provoke a withdrawal from participation, or conversely a greater motivation to gain some control of the consultation. Positive behaviours, such as being considerate or listening, appear to underpin stronger attachments between patients and professionals.

Patients' roles

In considering patients' roles in terms of human agency, the ways in which patients may be seen to engage actively in the consultation, as well as more passive forms of involvement, have been the topic of discussion throughout this book. By considering patients' roles as active or passive, it is possible, as shown in the chapters that analyse sequences from consultations, to distinguish between forms of participation and non-participation within any therapeutic context (see Chapter 7, for example). Further to this consideration of the nature of patients' contributions, Chapter 5 demonstrates how active participation of both the patient and the practitioner is a necessary component of homoeopathy, without which there is little chance of achieving a therapeutic relationship. Other examples have shown how the degree to which a patient is active or passive may depend on their desired level of responsibility. For example, Chapter 4 shows that patients may wish to have their doctor lead the consultation and determine the space available to participate, with the patients' responsibility being to articulate their problems clearly to facilitate the doctor's role. Chapter 3 reveals that, while passivity might be viewed in relation to a patient's lack of desire to be involved in a consultation, it might also illustrate an active detachment. This is paralleled by instances in actual consultations in which, through silence or refraining from talking, a patient conveys their resistance to a particular treatment option or proposal (see Extracts 2 and 3, Chapter 2; Stivers 2005a).

Patients' trust

The third variable relating to human agency concerns the patient's trust in the health professional. Trust is explicitly acknowledged to play a key part in the therapeutic process in homoeopathy, through its emphasis on rapport and empathy (Chapter 7). There is evidence in Chapter 4 that this is important for patients to feel they have a good consultation, including the need for professionals to admit when they lack knowledge, as in Extract 17. Chapter 3 also emphasizes the importance of trust in determining how involved patients wish to be in a consultation, with lack of trust being a motivator for wanting increased involvement (as found by Kraetschmer et al. 2004), and more involvement appearing to reinforce feelings of trust.

An overview of the holistic framework for understanding patient participation

The holistic framework of patient participation thus consists of three elements: components, levels and contexts. Figure 10.1 shows the matrix of interactions between components and levels. In addition, patient participation is a concept that can be understood along two dimensions. One dimension concerns patients' and health professionals' approaches to the health care consultation. The other dimension concerns the enactment of the health care consultation itself, in its sequential details, viewed along a continuum from 'non-involvement' to 'full dialogue'. Participation cannot easily be applied as a global term to describe a consultation, since it takes different forms in relation to different components. It is a dynamic concept that is likely to vary in level within and across consultations for any individual patient, and is contingent upon the contexts of structure and agency in which it is enacted. (See the Educational Supplement, p. 212).

COMPONENT	PATIENT'S LEVEL OF INVOLVEMENT				
	Non-involved 0	Information-seeking / receptive 1	Information-giving / dialogue 2	Shared decision-making 3	Autonomous decision-making 4
Contribution to action sequences					
Influence in problem definition					
Share in reasoning process					
Influence in decision-making					
Emotional reciprocity					

Figure 10.1 Matrix of interactions between components and levels of patient participation.

Would we recommend patient participation as a policy?

Given these complexities, if patient participation is to be recommended, it cannot be a blanket policy. It is clear that while some patients express a desire to have more voice within health care consultations, others do not. For those patients who want health professionals to make decisions on their behalf, it can be anxiety-provoking to be asked for their opinions. Doctors attempting to practise shared decision-making with patients who do not want to do so are likely to undermine these patients' confidence in their doctor, and erode their trust that the doctor knows what he or she is doing.

We have to ask who is advocating greater participation. Clearly the World Health Organization and some national *governments* are, but this is not true of all national governments. As discussed in Chapters 1 and 3, the motivations for these policies include both consumerist and democratic perspectives. We need to ask whether the metaphors of the market place or the political process are appropriate for the delivery of health care. Some would argue that, when experiencing illness and suffering, people do not want to be treated either as customers or as voters.

It is also apparent that many *researchers* are advocating greater participation. The health care communication research literature is increasingly organized around the degree to which patients actively participate in their encounters with health professionals (Cahill 1996; Little et al. 2001). As described in Chapter 1, the motivations of these researchers are manifold. For some, it has to do with achieving a better balance between the biomedical and disease context, on the one hand, and a more integrated illness context that incorporates the patient perspective on the other (Roter 2000; Sullivan 2003); achieving more humane and ethical practice (Mishler 1984); or the achievement of better outcomes (Coulter 1991; Street and Millay 2001). Others adopt a more political perspective that starts from the position that patients have the right to greater involvement in health care and that the evidence (such as it is) that this is associated with improved health care outcomes is a secondary consideration (Barnes 1997; Guadagnoli and Ward 1998; Hogg 1999).

We also need to ask whether there are any signs that *patients* themselves are seeking greater participation. The difficulty for patients is that many have no institutional affiliations with one another. There are exceptions to this in the form of self-help and other kinds of patient groups, usually disease-focused. Chapters 3 and 4 suggest that, in terms of information, some patients would like more information about their condition, and would also like practitioners to listen to them more. There is evidence that some patients would like to share decisions with practitioners, but by no means all of them. A few people want to be able to make their own decisions about their health care. If we are to be guided by patients' preferences, then it would seem that we can advocate more information exchange (more information given to patients and more attention paid to the things that patients want their practitioners to know about them), but that we would have to be more cautious in advocating shared or autonomous decision-making.

Although it seems that there is not a great deal of support, from either patients or practitioners, for patients to make autonomous decisions, a significant minority of people already do so. These include many people living with chronic conditions, as well as those who choose complementary and alternative medicine (CAM). For example, patients deciding to consult a CAM practitioner (when it is not something recommended by their doctor or nurse) are making autonomous decisions about the nature of their own treatment. These decisions are often not known to their orthodox practitioners, and if known, may not be approved of. Some people choose to consult a CAM practitioner precisely because they want a more mutual relationship. Thus, in conceptualizing the levels of participation in health care, we need to include the autonomous choices of individuals to seek treatment outside the orthodox health care system. The question of whether patients consulting CAM practitioners actually experience mutuality is an interesting one, as shown in Chapters 5 and 7. People may make an autonomous decision on the basis of their experience of orthodox medicine, but then find themselves engaging in non-participatory CAM consultations.

In Chapter 6, we argue that it is better to use research findings to raise awareness than to advocate greater participation. Moving straight from research findings to training programmes can have unexpected consequences when programmes fail to take account of the normative character of institutional interaction. Rather, we suggest that research findings can be used to raise the awareness of practitioners and help them reflect on their own practices. This awareness needs to take in the variations in participation according to particular consultation phases, individual differences in patients' preferences, understanding of the particular constraints and opportunities for participation across different health care settings and types of consultation, with different types of health professional. This makes the task of health professionals even more exacting and challenging than we first indicated in Chapter 1. Raising increased awareness of these dimensions in consultations, and of the complex issues that surround questions concerning patient participation, is the motivation behind the educational supplements relating to each chapter.

What remains less obvious is how these findings can be used to help patients manage their consultations with health care practitioners, and this is one of the challenges for policy-makers and researchers. We need to develop innovative methods of helping the users of health services to benefit from the findings of research if we are not to perpetuate the imbalance of knowledge and skills that characterize professional–patient interactions.

Institutional encounters such as health care consultations are governed by strong, often unarticulated rules. It can be argued that greater patient participation involves breaking these rules. Parsons' model of the sick role (1951) set out a normative framework of rights and obligations for both the sick person and the practitioner. While this model is applicable to certain situations and not others, the normative character of health care interactions remains in place. Some people may advocate patient participation precisely because they want to redress the balance of power between patients and professionals, and challenge medical dominance. Others may advocate patient participation because they feel that patients can have a greater voice within the existing framework and so improve the quality of care, with positive effects on health outcomes.

If we advocate patient participation, we should be clear about which of these scenarios we endorse. Whichever we choose, we need to keep in mind the fact that not all patients wish to participate in all situations and at all times, if at all. Whether active involvement at a minimal level incrementally leads to more positive endorsement of patient participation, and to willingness by patients to take increasing responsibility for the outcomes of participation, remains an open question.

How could patient participation be measured?

Although it might be thought that there is no need to measure patient participation, but rather to know what it is and whether it occurs within a consultation, some would argue that measurement offers a way to evaluate how effective any policy that promotes it might be (see Entwistle et al. 2004). Adopting this latter position, we offer some initial thoughts on how this might be accomplished and its potential utility to the various stakeholders. We recognize that a number of quantitative measures have already been developed to measure aspects of participation (Elwyn et al. 2003b) and the importance of concepts such as trust (Anderson and Dedrick 1990) and empathy (Mercer et al. 2004; Mercer and Howie 2006). However, in this book we have deliberately focused on a qualitative understanding of participation to draw out the complexities of the concept in a way that might underpin development of a more nuanced and context-specific set of measures.

Effective measurement needs to begin by understanding the concept itself, which has been the aim of these various investigations in the book. From here we can begin to identify those components (see pp. 180–1 above) that pertain to participation (or involvement). The matrix developed from the holistic framework (see Figure 10.1 above) allows us to consider both how patients and professionals wish to be involved and also to evaluate the positions that patients occupy, in relation to each of the components of patient participation in the consultation. A simple count of those occurrences as a proportion of all occurrences would produce a relative measure of participation, but would require definition of how much of the interaction counts as one 'unit' of potential participation.

When considering the interactional aspects of patient participation or potential participation, conversation analysis (CA) may be suitable. CA is a method that investigates the particulars of talk-in-interaction in order to find what sorts of things the participants of an encounter themselves treat as relevant, or as suitable ways to act in a specific context (such as a medical consultation). In Chapter 7, for instance, it was shown that patients interpret doctors' accounts of diagnosis as an opportunity for them to offer their own diagnostic suggestion. In short, with CA it is possible to show what sort of second actions usually follow a specific type of first action, what sort of third actions again follow the second actions, etc. Further, as CA is particularly apt for sequential analysis, it also provides tools to analyse the placement of activities in the overall structure (or course) of the encounter analysed.

To give an example of a possible application, one could separate the cases where the doctor follows the patient's initiative and discusses the topic evoked by the patient, and those where this does not happen. Further, one could examine the placement of the initial actions in the overall structural organization of the consultation and see whether there is a difference in the 'success' of a patient's initiatives in different phases of the consultation. These analyses could be carried out quantitatively in order to explore statistical relationships between variables (see e.g. Stivers 2005b).

The matrix presented in Figure 10.1 is intended to facilitate an examination of the interactive positions between professionals and patients within each component of the consultation. This matrix can be used to locate their respective desired levels of involvement within each component, prior to evaluating the resultant levels that patients find themselves in. For example, a patient might be happy for a professional to define the problem and inform the patient of their diagnosis (level 1), but wish to have dialogue with that professional in the reasoning process (level 2). On the other hand, while the professional might be happy to determine the problem and inform the patient of it (level 1), the professional might believe that there is no need for discussion of the reasoning process and effectively exclude the patient from it (level 0). We could conjecture that the resultant level of interaction in this example might be level 1 for the problem definition component. However, the component concerned with the reasoning process would be more contested and, depending on the relative power and willingness to accommodate the other party, the resultant level might be anywhere between levels 0 (adopting the professional's preference) and 2 (adopting the patient's preference). Figure 10.2 illustrates how the matrix presented earlier in Figure 10.1 might be used in this example.

We could further attempt to isolate specific patient actions in a particular context that might indicate what level of involvement is being pursued by a patient. For example, we might identify a first position act or resistance to a professional's agenda in the reasoning process, from which we might deduce that the patient wanted to be at level 2, due to showing signs of wanting to give their understanding of the diagnosis. We would need to be careful that we did not assume that such actions could always be interpreted in this way, since it would depend on the particular context of the interaction.

Further refinements in the measurement process could lead to scales of

	Non-involved 0	Information-seeking/receptive 1	Information-giving/Dialogue 2
Influence in problem definition		Patient-desired involvement Professional-desired involvement of patient	
Outcome		X	
Share in reasoning process	Professional-desired involvement of patient		Patient-desired involvement
Outcome	?	?	?

Figure 10.2 Examples of interactions between specific components and levels of patient participation.

participation. One example would be to develop measures of the extent to which participation is contingent or constituted by the interaction, as sketched in Figure 10.3. This illustrates how we might conceive of differences in patient participation between types of medical practice, on a continuum from participation being contingent on the components of interaction through to where participation is constituted by them. In the three examples of medical practice, discussed in Chapter 7, we might place allopathic medicine as typically lying at the contingent end of the spectrum and psychoanalysis at the other, with homoeopathy occupying a position somewhere in between. A comparative framework such as this opens up possibilities for drawing on the professional stocks of interaction (SIKs) of different therapeutic styles to understand, and potentially promote, effective patient participation.

Another possibility would be to develop scales of the degree or intensity of participation, through measuring the level of involvement which patients

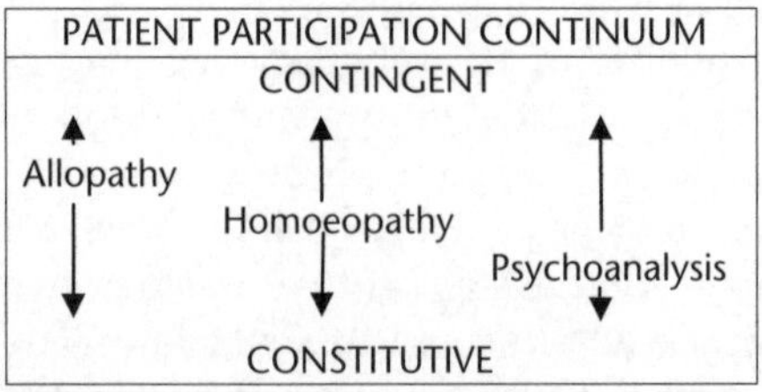

Figure 10.3 The contingent-constitutive dimension of participation.

reach, while bearing in mind that 'more' participation is not necessarily desired or effective. If we were able to develop such a measure, then we would be in a position to evaluate the effect of the various contextual variables on participation through some form of asymmetric statistical modelling. The outcome of this could lead to recommendations as to how to influence the desired degree of participation in the most effective and efficient way.

What else do we need to know about patient participation?

While the studies presented in this book offer an array of examples of patient participation, and provide insights into the processes that shape participation, there are clearly many contexts which have been little explored, and others that have not been mentioned. In this last section we briefly sketch in some of these gaps.

First, in studies reported elsewhere, health professionals' communication styles have been shown to influence the ways in which patients participate in health consultations (for example, Collins et al. 2005). Second, although lack of time is in itself insufficient explanation for restrictions on patient participation, it does play a part. A further related structural aspect may be the extent to which the services are public or private, in which time can be a key variable.

In relation to socio-demographic influences, patient and health professional characteristics of age, gender and ethnicity, for example, are expected to show distinct relationships with some of the interactive features of consultations, such as the changing expectations over the life course of an individual. A number of other patient characteristics might influence the way in which a consultation evolves. Chapter 3 refers to a number of possible influences on the likely demand for involvement by patients, such as the patient's educational level, or their degree of confidence. Other aspects of personality, such as the emotional disposition to illness, may impinge on the patient–professional interaction.

Another potentially interesting line of investigation concerns patients' strategic goals for the consultation. Some of these goals will be related to the institutional tasks and roles, while others will reflect patients' roles and expectations of the consultation.

One final area to be considered in further research is the role of third parties to the consultation. Virtually all the research shown here is focused on a dyadic relationship between one patient and one health care professional in a consultation. Many consultations occur with other parties present, whether carers, family members or friends, or other health professionals in a multidisciplinary team: all of whom also influence the opportunities for patient participation.

Conclusion

Patient participation is a much more complex concept than is generally understood and certainly more so than current policies that promote it would suggest. The contributions of this book provide multiple entry points for seeing what patient participation looks like in practice and how our understanding of it can be developed through further focused and nuanced research. The chapters in this book allow us to consider patient participation from two viewpoints: in ideal form, through the eyes of patients and professionals, and in terms of how it is actually enacted and may be observed, between patients and professionals in their communication within real consultations.

A range of methods has been used to explore these interactions, using conversation analysis of recorded consultations, as well as analysis of verbatim accounts of interviews and focus groups. The analytical methods we have used are exclusively qualitative, since our enquiries have been descriptive, exploratory and interpretative in character. The aim has been to develop an understanding of participation as it occurs in practice. Given the insights this book has contributed to the study of patient participation, we have suggested a framework that might assist in the task of quantifying the concept, should this be felt necessary. However, in general, we remain sceptical about the possibility or even the value of attempting to make generalizations about participation in health care consultations as a whole.

In conclusion, we encourage readers of this book to engage critically with the ideas and analyses presented in it. We hope that readers will draw on their own experiences, beliefs, research or practice, to consider how far this book helps to understand and develop the concept of patient participation. We offer a series of exercises in the educational supplement to each chapter (see pp. 197–212) which we hope will make this task easier and most fruitful. Undoubtedly much remains to be understood in this highly topical and important field of enquiry. We hope that the framework we have constructed will facilitate future developments in practice, teaching and research.

Recommendations: summary

- Participation can be understood in terms of components, levels and contexts.
- A distinction should be made between desired and achieved levels of participation.

- Participation cannot be understood in global terms but only in relation to specific settings and types of consultations.
- Attempts to measure patient participation or to evaluate its outcomes need to begin with, and remain sensitive to, an understanding of the contextual influences and interactional processes that influence its forms.

Afterword

Encounters with health care: a personal viewpoint

Anon

It's human nature to want to be perceived by others as interesting, and as flawless physically and mentally. So to have strangers ask you personal questions, and perhaps also do things to your body, is in effect like having your social armour attacked.

I don't like being watched. This makes my thoughts go blank. To undergo a medical examination or consultation is probably one of my least favourite experiences. Coupled with this blankness, I seem to go into an unhelpful polite mode. I wait to be asked a question, and I won't interrupt with some relevant symptom or fact. So this important information tends to float off and dissolve into my blank state of thoughts. In consultations, this creates a time delay in my thought processes. I don't think of questions until it's too late and I've left the consultation.

This, I know, is quite a common reaction. When a friend of mine was told that her tumour was benign, she was so shocked and elated that she didn't really register anything else during the rest of the consultation. All she knew was that it wasn't cancer and she'd have more appointments for further tests; but afterwards, she couldn't recount exactly what these tests would be for, or what else had been said.

Once, in a hospital waiting room, an elderly woman next to me knew that she would be asked to put a gown on before her consultation. In a whisper she asked me if I thought she would have to remove her underwear. This seems such a simple thing, but she was highly agitated and said she hadn't slept for worrying about it. We cornered a nurse who explained what was necessary, and this woman did seem to calm down. Maybe if she had been given a little more information before or during her wait, she would have been in a calmer and more receptive state of mind for the consultation ahead.

I recently underwent some procedures to rid me of a condition I'd detested and tried to hide since childhood. Half of me felt overjoyed and hugely grateful that this was about to happen, but decades of secrecy and shame are hard to publicize; so the other half of me was still the frightened and sad little girl who cringed when my condition, the treatment procedure, and the prognosis were continually – or so it seemed – being broadcast to the whole ward and its visitors by at least 12 members of staff who were just doing their jobs and consulting with me, in my curtained area. This was my first experience of being in hospital. I was shocked to be treated as one of a stream of patients on the ward's conveyer belt. It struck me as odd that the nurses and doctors didn't see the need for privacy when to me the condition had been so hugely unmentionable for so long. I couldn't help wondering why they didn't speak a little more quietly behind the thin curtains; did they have to shout so? All these factors prevented me from being able to talk about my concerns during those procedures, and I was left with unvoiced and unanswered questions.

When my newborn baby was rushed to casualty, I was stunned by the urgency and forcefulness of the medical team. I knew the invasive procedures were vital and so, although frightened I watched carefully and answered questions as they were fired at me. But my partner, who also understood the urgency, and who is normally calm and laid back, became increasingly agitated. His shock and feelings of hopelessness meant he couldn't witness the scene. A brilliant nurse took us to one side and explained what was happening, her attitude was incredibly calming, and although very young, and childless herself, she delivered her empathy perfectly. Her actions helped us to become involved; I actually believed that she could understand how we both felt, and we were soon reunited with a poorly but stable baby.

Health professionals' life experiences are often short, sheltered and very different compared to those of many of their patients. And in the limited time they have, for a consultation or to perform some medical or nursing procedure, it must be hard, though not impossible, to imagine the patient's views and feelings, and to judge their reactions to being ill, and to all that this will entail.

In an ideal world, medical consultations would be unrushed, and take place in a soothing environment. They would be more like the homoeopathic consultations I have attended, where I almost feel better simply because someone is taking their time to create a picture of the whole of me. This, in turn, makes me feel understood, and able to express my thoughts.

From a patient's point of view, so that we are able to feel involved and to take a more active part, any health professional, as well as their medical knowledge, needs to have patience, diplomacy, and even telepathic skills, but, above all, empathy. Maybe this could be injected; their natural supply must run thin on occasions during their careers.

I began reading through the chapters in this book as I started my own nursing training. I've found there is much to learn from reading about different health care situations in which people find themselves. And the details of words used, the tone of voice, how respect for the patient is shown, a calm attitude; these all play their part. In the light of my own experiences, involving patients is going to be a continual challenge – something to keep practising and to keep thinking about.

Educational Supplements

Introduction

Each of the exercises and questions here can be considered from the viewpoint of one's own health care experiences, whether these relate to being a patient and/or a health professional; a carer; a citizen; someone designing a research project; or a manager of a health care clinic or surgery. The supplements can be used from any perspective – by members of voluntary organizations and patient groups; by health professionals, whether trainee or qualified; by students of language and communication; by researchers in health and social sciences; and by educators who are designing courses in communication and consultation skills. Each supplement involves a combination of individual and group learning, and covers a range of discussion topics and activities to stimulate learning and debate on themes relating to patient participation. It is not generally necessary to have read a chapter first, in order to be able to complete the exercises (except in the case of Chapter 6, where reading the chapter provides a definition of 'formulations'). The reader may even prefer to begin with the supplements, as a route into the chapters.

Supplement to Chapter 1 Understanding the process of patient participation

Learning more about patient participation

1. In relation to the material presented in Chapter 1, consider the following questions, either by writing your own notes, or in discussion with colleagues. You can then use your responses to guide your reading of this book.
   (a) When you think about patient participation, what does it mean to you?
   (b) What do you expect to learn from this book?
   (c) On the basis of reading Chapter 1, what particular questions do you have (e.g. in relation to your practice, in supporting your staff)?

Now take a perspective different to the one you have adopted (for example, if you are a health professional, now take the perspective of a patient, or of a researcher). Consider what kinds of questions, viewpoints or motivations that person might have for learning about patient participation.

2 Use the quotes below, or find others from the literature, to discuss what each one reflects about:
   (a) The kinds of positions given to patients and health professionals.
   (b) The rights and responsibilities placed on patients and health professionals.

   In each quote:

   (c) Whose perspective is being adopted?
   (d) What effect does this perspective have on your understanding and interpretation of the points being made?
   (e) What does the quote say about patient participation?

Quote A

By the same institutional definition the sick person is not, of course competent to help himself, or what he can do is, except for trivial illness, not adequate. But in our culture there is a special definition of the kind of help he needs, namely, professional, technically competent help. The nature of this help imposes a further disability or handicap upon him. He is not only generally not in a position to do what needs to be done, but he does not 'know' what needs to be done or how to do it. It is not merely that he, being bedridden, cannot go down to the drugstore to get what is needed, but that he would, even if well, not be qualified to do what is needed, and to judge what needs to be done. There is, that is to say, a 'communication gap'.

(Parsons 1951: 441)

Quote B

In a patient-centred approach, the health professional: . . . explores the patient's main reason for the visit, concerns, and need for information, seeks an integrated understanding of the patient's world – that is, their whole person, emotional needs, and life issues, finds common ground on what the problem is and mutually agrees on management, enhances prevention and health promotion, and enhances the continuing relationship between patient and doctor.

(Stewart 2001: 445)

Quote C

We conceive of the consultation as a meeting between one person who has, by his training and by his experience, access to scarce and specialist knowledge and another who has, by experience, immersion in his culture and past discussion, a set of ideas about what is happening to him. Both parties form models of what is wrong, what should be done, what are the consequences of the problem, its treatment and so on, based on their own reasoning and background knowledge. These models may involve a degree of inconsistency and uncertainty. A major aim of the consultation, then, is the initiation of a process of explicit sharing of models, so that the patient is placed in a situation, as far as he wants to be, where he can choose to take advantage of the specialist biomedical ideas and skills his medical adviser can offer.

(Tuckett et al. 1985: 217)

Supplement to Chapter 2 Methods for studying patient participation

Exploring different methods and research perspectives in the study of patient participation

This exercise is presented in two parts. The first part involves working individually, and the second part involves working as a group.

Three linked extracts are provided for the purposes of this exercise. Extract A is from a consultation between a doctor and a patient who has diabetes. Extracts B and C are from semi-structured interviews following that same consultation, which involved viewing video-recorded clips from the consultation. Extract B is from the interview with the doctor, and Extract C is from the interview with the patient.

You might want to repeat this exercise using your own or your students' data, or using extracts provided in the other chapters in this book.

Part I Working on your own

1 Taking each of the extracts below in turn, read through the extract and, considering only the information in that one extract, make notes about what this extract tells you, regarding how health professionals and patients who have diabetes might approach a discussion about diet and lifestyle issues.

2 Still working on your own, now compare and contrast the different extracts and your notes about each of them. In particular, consider what is added by each perspective of this consultation situation as represented in your notes, as you collate them. Does the combination of perspectives presented in the different data sources add more than if only one data source was used? And, if so, what is added, and why?

Extract A From a consultation between a doctor and a patient who has diabetes (D = doctor; P = patient)

```
 1  D:  .hhh right so: um: you've been trying thuh diet now
 2      since (.) it's for three months really
 3  P:  Mm
 4  D:  Urm: (.) an it actually did bring things down tuh
 5      start with
 6      (0.5)
 7  D:  Erm: but its actually gone up a little bit which
 8      er[:
 9  P:    [ri:ght
10  D:  Not much it was from nine point one last time up tuh
11      nine point five this time so. hh it's not a great
12      increase but uh- I think that shows probably that's
13      as good as diet is gonna do for you
14  P:  R[i::ght]
15  D:   [ .h h ]Erm: an I think when:[: :, ]
16  P:                                [I thi]nk I probably
17      (0.5)
18  P:  Relaxed a bit there as w[ell   i]n fairness[ so: ]I=
19  D:                          [Ri:ght]           [right]
20  P:  =think I can: bring thuh diet back a bit more
21  D:  Ri:ght okay (.) .hh
22      (0.5)
23  D:  How duh yuh feel about that then becau:se um::
24      (1.4)
25  D:  If yuh feel that you could perhaps be a bit tighter
26      on yuh diet prepared tuh give things another month or
27      so before we will consider tablets
        ((29 lines omitted in which the patient reminds the doctor
        that he is already on a small dose))
57  D:  =D'yuh- think instead of cre- >increasing that up
58      then it would be better tuh<
59      (0.5)
60  D:  P'raps
61      (0.9)
62  D:  Try a bit more: harder with thuh diet[ or: ]
63  P:                                       [I thi]nk so
64      for thuh [nex]t month ce[rtainly ]
65  D:           [Yeh]          [next mon]th uh so yeh=
66  P:  =We godda-um: meeting with thuh dietician:
67      later this month=
68  D:  =Ri:ght
```

P: An: erm (0.7) I lost a bit then put a bit back but I
think I'm down again no[w I l]ost a bit on holiday
D: [ri:ght]
as[well]
D: [righ]t hm=
P: =s[o:: e]r it[sh]ould be alright over
D: [right] [hm]
thuh thuh next few weeks
D: Fine ok[ay]
P: [So]: an I need tuh lose weight anyway so
D: Yeah (0.4) yeh a mean yuhknow thuh-a think given th-
:- maybe as yuh c- as yuh weight comes down thuh
requirements fuh thuh tablets will completely
disappear . . .

(Consultation between GP and patient with diabetes, B-117-329)

Extract B From a semi-structured interview with the doctor who took part in the consultation above (R = researcher; D = doctor)

R: Yes, so, the diet. Would you, 'cause you don't really with
him, follow up what exactly he's eating or whatever and I
was wondering whether that's something you <u>would</u> do with
some patients or not or?
D: I tend not to for the simple reason is that, you know, again
when they first get diagnosed, they, we give them a leaflet
and a diet sheet so that they've got all the stuff on there.
And we refer them to the dieticians as well. And then the
dieticians give them more information. So they're getting
information from elsewhere and when the nurses see them in
the week before, the nurses talk about diet with them. So
you know they are getting information from diet on three
sources and I don't really see my expertise really is in
that field. So I tend not to do anything about them. I mean,
if somebody
comes in and says, 'I'm drinking 15 pints of beer a day',
I'll say, 'well you know that's not good when you're
diabetic. Try and drink dry white wine instead or
something.' ((Laughter))
R: Yeah, yeah. So it's not an area that <u>you</u> feel that <u>you</u>
need to cover.
D: Because it's covered by other people.

(Semi-structured interview with GP, D–117)

Extract C From a semi-structured interview with the patient in Extract A

```
If I were dealing with this and not [my doctor], I think I would be more brutal, in a way. But what we're really doing at the moment is 'you're ignoring the problem, and I'm giving you the tablets to ease it'. And [if it were me] 'I'd say really you should be doing more, you know it's your problem, it's not my problem . . .' In fairness it's my problem not [the doctor's]. He's my guide. But the ownership is with me. Because it's true isn't it, no matter what medication he puts me on, unless I get my bit right it won't go away.
```

(Semi-structured interview with patient with diabetes, D–329)

Part II Working as a group

Now that you have considered each extract on its own merits, form small groups to discuss your findings:

1. Compare your findings with those of others in your group. What are the differences and similarities in your perspectives on and interpretations of these data? Why might these differences and similarities exist?
2. Consider your own responses to having your findings challenged by the group, and to having to challenge the findings of others.
3. What sort of evidence for practice does this exercise yield?
4. What do you think are the dangers and disadvantages of trying to reach a consensus with such diverse data and methods? What are the strengths and advantages?

Supplement to Chapter 3 The meaning of patient involvement and participation in health care consultations

Health professional and patient experiences of involvement: exercises in reflection, role play and group discussion.

This role play activity was first described in Thompson (1999).

Part I Working individually

Think back to a recent health care consultation, or, if this is too distant or has never occurred, think of a similar communication situation, such as a one-to-one meeting between a student and their teacher, or a performance review between an employee and their employer. Try to think how you wanted to involve yourself (or not) as a patient/student, or how as a health professional/teacher you wanted to involve the patient/student. Which level of involvement seems to best fit what you wanted, and which level did you occupy in the event? What seemed to be important in deciding which level resulted? If the levels of involvement varied during the consultation you are thinking of, choose one part of it where it would be appropriate to think about one level.

Part II Working as a group

Divide the group into roughly equal numbers of 'patients' (or 'students') and 'health professionals' (or 'teachers'). Then divide each of these broad groupings into three sub-groups based on their preferred style of involvement:

1 Patients/students
   (a) Submissive/passive
   (b) Shared decision-makers
   (c) Autonomous decision-makers.
2 Health professionals/teachers
   (a) Paternalists
   (b) Shared decision-makers
   (c) Informants (not decision-makers) of professional knowledge.

Imagine that the professionals are working in one of three practices (e.g. health centre, hospital, university department), each featuring the style listed above. The patients/students seek an imaginary consultation (about whatever relevant topic they like) and proceed from one practice to another, experiencing the three different styles in turn.

Part III Discussion

Participants should then discuss how the different consultations worked, which one they preferred, and what they liked and disliked about each combination of their own style with that of the other party, i.e. each person will have three consultation experiences to report on.

Supplement to Chapter 4 What is a good consultation and what is a bad one?

Evaluating patients' and carers' experiences of involvement in consultations

The theme of Chapter 4 – what is 'good' and 'bad' about consultations from the patient's point of view – can be explored in more depth through one or more of the following activities.

1 Everyone is asked to bring particular experiences of good or bad consultations to the session (either their own or those of a family

member, or friend) and to be prepared to discuss them. It might be useful to have spent some time before the session writing these down.

2 Rerun the research on which this chapter is based in small groups during the session. Begin the activity by collecting, through a brainstorming or other activity, the features of a good or a bad consultation. The ideas are then collated and discussed with reference to how they relate to the idea of participation in consultations, with particular reference to the academic literature, policy documents, and/or information from patient organizations.

3 Prior to the session, and perhaps prior to reading Chapter 4, students could interview people about their views and experiences of features of 'good' and 'bad' consultations. In the session, students feed back the insights gathered. The themes and ideas generated could then be considered in the context of policy and research relating to participation.

4 Either as a means of introducing the themes of Chapter 4 prior to reading it, or facilitating further discussion following it, additional material could be supplied about good/bad consultations and used to listen to or read about patients'/carers' experiences and views on this subject. The material might be stories in newspapers, videos, television programmes, or films. Two useful sources of such material are the DIPEx database (DIPEx: Personal Experiences of Health and Illness: www.dipex.org) and *Cinemeducation* (Alexander et al. 2005).

5 On the basis of selected material (as suggested in 4), students can be asked to critique a particular health care experience, and to distil what did or didn't work.

The discussions and activities suggested above could also be based on review of and reflection on 'good' or 'bad' teaching and learning experiences.

Supplement to Chapter 5 A feeling of equality

Building mutuality in the opening phases of consultations

Consider these two examples of opening phases, from different types of consultation.

Extract A (H = homoeopath; P = patient)

```
H:  So (0.3) lets talk about your chest.
    (0.6)
P:  Right. ^hhh.
H:  .h This cough
P:  .hh Yes (0.5) I notice when this: (0.9) I- I don't think
```

it's been a hundred percent since I (.) I had the
operation because I'm on the anaesthetic=
H: =Right=
P: =Right. hh but (.) It was a bonus because I got through
anaesthetic-s that was my-[.h
H: [Did you take phosphorus
(0.5)
P: .hh (0.2) erm (0.2) [yes
H: [Did you end up ta[king phosphorus
P: [Yes, yes I did (.)
I did. hh because the did lots of checks on my chest n: I
had to do a breathing test n they put oxygen on me
straight away n.hhh I did think they would do the operation
I was quite chesty n I was thinking ^don't cough ^don't
cough.

(Video-recorded consultation in homoeopathy, B-101-341)

Extract B (D = doctor; P = patient)

P: Morning Doctor<
(.)
D: HELLO THERE
(3.4)
P: ehhhh How're you
(0.3)
D: I'm alright?
(1.0)
D: How're you.
P: Eh not so ↑bad actually
D: Good, good,
(0.4)
D: How's [your voi:ce been]
P: [( )]
(0.6)
P: (eez) what Do[c t o r?]
D: [How's your] voi:ce been.
'Bout the s[a :m e]
P: ['S ↑al-:r]ight yeh it's
j['s (s'same)
D: [(Ri:ght,)
(.)
D: Okay
(0.7)
D: Well the ↑SCAN that we did, (0.4) ↓Ah:. (1.4) I got the<

(1.4) the la:st little< (0.4) s:ynopsis bit b't this
shows the rest'v it,
(10.5)
D: °↓Right.°
(0.3)
D: °↓O-okay°
(2.8)
D: Well I think that uh:m (1.6) the cee tee scan s'↑por:ts:
the diagnosis, of it being an ear↓ly (0.3) tumor in- (.)
in the voi:ce↓box.
P: Eyeh.
(.)
D: So:< (0.2) I think that, fr'm that point'v view I know
that you were never very keen on (1.1) surgery anyway
but I think that (.) the chances of radio therapy
(0.5) cur↓ingthis are,↓ very good.=

(Video-recorded consultation in head and neck cancer, B-102-357)

1 For each case, consider:
   (a) Do you think mutuality is present?
   (b) If so, how is it being shown?
   (c) Can you identify ways in which the health professional and patient are *building* this mutuality?
   (d) If you do not think mutuality is present, how is mutuality being blocked?
   (e) How might the opening be adapted by the health professional to promote mutuality?
2 What are your own experiences of mutuality, rapport and empathy in consultations?
3 Do you think these are qualities which can be taught? If so, what teaching/learning methods do you think would be most effective?

Supplement to Chapter 6 Patient participation in formulating and opening sequences

Identifying formulations and exploring their uses in consultations

1 The students select videos or audio recordings of consultations to work with. These may be recordings of their own consultations, of colleagues' consultations, or recordings made for research purposes. There are also a number of video publications available, such as Denning and Draper (2004).

2 The students work through the data, noting formulations used by the health professionals and by their patients. For each formulation, students identify whether it is a formulating summary or an action formulation.
3 The students then:
   (a) Describe, by observing whole sequences, the cognitive and organizational functions of the observed formulations.
   (b) Look for any indications that formulating summaries are being challenged or resisted by patients.
   (c) Seek out inappropriate use of action formulations by the doctor, in situations where there was no prior agreement about the course of action.
   (d) Discuss the consequences of all the above for patients' participation and for health professionals' training.

Supplement to Chapter 7 What is patient participation?

Types of encounter, key activities, and opportunities for patients' participation

1 Consider the differences and similarities between two or more of the following types of encounter:

Type of encounter	*Examples in this book*
Nurse–patient encounter	Chapter 8
General practice consultation	Chapters 6 and 7, and Exercise for Chapter 2
Homoeopathic consultation	Chapters 5 and 7
Psychoanalytic encounter	Chapter 7
Surgeon–patient consultation in hospital out-patients clinic	Exercises for Chapters 5 and 9

   (a) What is the purpose of the encounter?
   (b) What are the key activities necessary to fulfil its purpose?
   (c) How do each of these key activities influence the nature of patients' and health professionals' contributions, and the ways in which patient participation can be realized?
   (d) What differences do you observe, or might you anticipate, in relation to patients' contributions across the different types of encounter and key activities?

2 Look at videos of medical consultations, or, if possible, record your own consultation (or alternatively, one-to-one tutorial or similar), and bring it to the session. Locate the section where diagnosis and/or treatment decision and response to it are given. Consider the opportunities the patient has to give their opinion on the diagnosis or treatment decision. How do these opportunities influence what the patient can say, and how they can contribute? Could there be more opportunities for patient participation? If so, how could the health professional enhance the patient's opportunities?

Supplement to Chapter 8 Nursing assessments and other tasks

Structuring opportunities for patient participation in nurse consultations

1 On the basis of the presented data, design an opening (its components, and possible phrasings) for:
   (a) the admissions interview;
   (b) the diabetes review consultation;
   (c) the specialist nurse consultation that follows on from the doctor's.
2 Use the example of the opening of a surgeon consultation, presented in the supplement to Chapter 5, to discuss the organizational constraints that can present themselves in the specialist cancer nurse consultation that follows. Consider how, in that nurse consultation, these constraints can be managed in such a way as to open up opportunities for the patient's participation.
3 Design a nursing assessment form, on paper, that offers flexibility and creativity in managing the admissions interview, in such a way as to encourage the patient's participation.
4 The following are a series of exercises which could be enacted through discussion and writing, with role play, and/or with simulated patients.
   (a) Imagine you are manager of the ward on which Extracts 2 and 7 in Chapter 8 took place. From your position as manager, consider for each extract: What could happen next? How would you re-organize the situation? What would you do next as manager? How would you advise/direct your nurses who are conducting these interviews? Explore the alternatives.
   (b) Either design your own situation/scenario for a patient who has newly arrived on the ward, or use Extract A from our data, presented below. Write the first scenes of the situation, in such a way as to reflect factors that restrict these patients' participation. Then

consider the same questions as in (a) above, from a manager's viewpoint.

Extract A is from a conversation between a registered nurse and William Evans, a 70-year-old retired gentleman who is being admitted into hospital for investigations into a suspected heart condition. As a Health Care Support worker escorts Mr Evans to the six-bedded ward and his bed space, she tells him that the nurse 'looking after' him will be along shortly to 'admit him'. As Mr Evans settles into the ward, a doctor appears, and tells Mr Evans that she will be along to 'clerk' him later in the morning and that they will have a chat about things then. As the doctor leaves, a nurse arrives and introduces herself as the person looking after him, she also states that she would like to ask him some questions as part of the 'assessment'. The patient sits down on a chair, and the nurse sits down on the bed behind a table:

Extract A (N = nurse: P patient)

```
N:  Hi William I'm Cath who's going to be looking after you
    today=
P:  ok ((laughs briefly))
N:  I uh (.) need to ask some questions to do the assessment
    so I'll do that now if that's ok
P:  yes that ok
    ((patient and nurse sit down))
N:  ok this shouldn't take too long now (.) just uh
    (21.0)   ((nurse reads the medical notes and writes))
N:  there are some things here ((points to medical notes))
    that I need to cover with you
P:  ((nods))
N:  so when were you last in hospital . . .
```

(Audio-recorded hospital admissions interview, 2087/LB)

Supplement to Chapter 9 Components of participation in health care consultations

Designing and critiquing research on patient participation

1 In relation to patient participation, think of some possible research questions that either you would like to investigate, or that you would like someone else to research. Select one of these research questions, and design a research setting and methods for studying your question, drawing upon the summary of the components of participation provided in Chapter 9.

2 In relation to your experiences and understandings of patient participation in health care consultation (from a personal and/or a professional viewpoint), design at least two critical questions to appraise the model of five key components of patient participation presented in Chapter 9.

3 As reported in Chapter 9, patients' initiatory actions have been little studied, but are significant in considering how patients can participate in shaping their care. In an unpublished paper on patients' initiatives in raising new concerns, Paul Drew describes how, beyond descriptions in the literature of how the interview format of the consultation restricts patients' participation, 'patients can initiate more radical departures from the medical agenda, by introducing matters which were not solicited by any question by the doctor'.

4 The following extract, from a consultation between a surgeon and a patient with laryngeal cancer, is an example of a patient initiative. With reference to this extract, consider the following questions:

(a) In what kind of environment are these patient initiatives launched?
(b) What are the design features of the turns containing these patient initiatives?
(c) How does the doctor respond in each case?
(d) What methods could you use to explore further the concerns raised by these patients?
(e) How would you design a study to research patients' initiatives?
(f) What recommendations would you make to doctors, so that patients' initiatives and the concerns they raise can find a place, be recognized, and be responded to?

The surgeon has been explaining that after a series of inconclusive tests, the most recent biopsy has confirmed cancer 'sitting right next to your voice box', which, he recommends, should be taken out as soon as possible (involving a tracheotomy). When the doctor has evidently come to the end of telling the patient the diagnostic news, and his recommended treatment, the patient 'interjects' with quite different matters, the problems he's been having with his sinus (lines 11–16) and earache (line 19). The sequence containing the patient initiative (lines 13–24) is highlighted.

Extract A (D = doctor: P = patient)

```
D:  I think that. hhhhhhh (.) uhm, hhh (0.4) in some
    respects, hhhhh (0.6) it- that's, a very good
    situation on which to be: because it means that if
    there's a small (local)ized area? (0.4) then:: (.)
    we c'n get it sorted out very °effectively°
```

(0.5)
D: An' I (.) I think (.) we might (.) it might
well be that if we take a lump out up (he:re. h we
might well find that there's nothing (led gon) up
here. .hh But I think that (.) you know we shouldn'
take any risks.
(1.7)
P: **h'M 'aving eh:: (0.2) (still having problem**
with the other (.) thing as well with thee (.)
(sinus problem. .hhh An' it °ih it e:ven seem to,
(.) irritate, (.) the work that you've done it by
hhh s-(stuff runnin' down seems
to. hh[h
D: [(Ri[ght
P: **[aggravate it °but°**
D: Ri:ght
(0.4)
P: **hAn:d uh-havin' a little trouble with ear a:che**
as we:ll,
(.)
D: .h Oka:y? Well [I'll (haa-)]
P: [He s o r t]'v handed me over
because this w'z [more u r g e]n[t,
D: [I t i : s] [Ah well this i:s.
uh this is. [We need t]o get on an' get that sorted
P: [(Mmhm?)]
D: ou:[t and, I think==that uh:m (0.7) it would be
P: [(Mm)
advisable f'r us to: um ask the radiotherapist as
we:ll.

(Video-recorded consultation in head and neck cancer, B-359-133)

Supplement to Chapter 10 An integrative approach to patient participation in consultations

Using a holistic framework to review and assess experiences of participation

1 Think of a recent consultation you experienced (either as a professional or patient). Using Figure 10.1 (see p. 185), reflect on how either you (if you are/were a patient) or your patient (if you are a professional) wanted to be involved (at which level) in each component.
2 How did you try to achieve this level?

3 At which level did you feel you were actually involved in each component?
4 If this actual level was different to what you wanted, why do you think this was?

Appendix
Transcript Notation for Conversation Analysis

The relative timing of utterances

Intervals either within or between turns shown thus (0.7).

A discernible pause which is too short to be timed mechanically is shown as a micro-pause, thus (.).

Overlaps between utterances are indicated by square brackets, the point of overlap onset being marked with a single left-hand bracket.

Contiguous utterances, where there is no discernible interval between turns, are linked by an equals sign. Also used to indicate very rapid movement from one unit in a turn to the next.

Characteristics of speech delivery

Various aspects of speech delivery are captured in these transcripts by punctuation symbols (which, therefore, are not used to mark conventional grammatical units) and other forms of notation, as follows:

- a period indicates a falling intonation;
- a comma indicates a continuing intonation;
- a question mark indicates a rising inflection (not necessarily a question).

The stretching of a sound is indicated by colons, the number of which correspond to the length of the stretching.

.h indicates inhalation, the length of which is indicated by the number of h's.

h. indicates outbreath, the length of which is indicated by the number of h's.

(hh) Audible aspirations are indicated in the speech in which they occur (including in laughter).

°° Degree signs indicate word(s) spoken very softly or quietly.

Sound stress is shown by italics, those words or parts of a word which are emphasized being underlined.

Particularly emphatic speech, usually with raised pitch, is shown by capital letters.

If what is said is unclear or uncertain, that is placed in parentheses.

See Jefferson (1984) for full details of this notation system.

References

Acheson, D. (1998) *Independent Inquiry into Inequalities and Health Report*. London: The Stationery Office.

Adams, T. (2001) The conversational and discursive construction of community psychiatric nursing for chronically confused people and their families, *Nursing Inquiry*, 8: 98–107.

Alexander, M., Lenahan, P. and Pavlov, A. (eds) (2005) *Cinemeducation*. Oxford: Radcliffe Publishing Ltd.

Alford, R.R. (1975) *Health Care Politics*. Chicago: University of Chicago Press.

Anderson, L.A. and Dedrick, R.F. (1990) Development of the trust in physician scale: a measure to assess interpersonal trust in patient–physician relationships. *Psychological Reports*, 67: 1091–100.

Arksey, H. and Knight, P. (1999) *Interviewing for Social Scientists*. London: Sage.

Armstrong-Esther, C., Browne, K.D. and McAfee, J.G. (1994) Elderly patients: still clean and sitting quietly, *Journal of Advanced Nursing*, 19: 264–71.

Arnstein, S.R. (1969) A ladder of citizen participation, *Journal of the American Institute of Planners*, 35(4): 216–24.

Ashworth, P. (1980) *Care to Communicate. An Investigation into Problems of Communication between Patients and Nurses in Intensive Therapy Units*. London: Royal College of Nursing.

Austin, J.L. (1962) *How to Do Things with Words*. Oxford: Clarendon Press.

Bales, R. (1951) *Interaction Process Analysis*. Cambridge: Addison-Wesley.

Balint, M. (1957) *The Doctor, the Patient, and the Illness*. London: Pitman Medical.

Ball, D.W. (1967) An abortion clinic ethnography, *Social Problems*, 14(3): 293–302.

Barbour, R. (1998) Mixing qualitative methods: quality assurance or qualitative quagmire?, *Qualitative Health Research*, 8: 352–61.

Barbour, R. (1999) The case for combining qualitative and quantitative approaches in health services research, *Journal of Health Services Research and Policy*, 4: 39–43.

Barnes, M. (1997) *Care, Communities and Citizens*. Harlow: Addison-Wesley Longman.

Barratt, J. (2005) A case study of styles of patient self-presentation in the nurse practitioner primary health care consultation, *Primary Health Care Research and Development*, 6: 327–38.

Barrett, R. (1988) Clinical writing and the documentary construction of schizophrenia, *Culture, Meaning and Psychiatry*, 12: 265–99.

Barry, C.A., Stevenson, F.A., Britten, N., Barber, N., Bradley, C.P. (2001) Giving voice to the lifeworld. More effective, more humane care? A qualitative study of doctor–patient communication in general practice, *Social Science and Medicine*, 53: 487–505.

Barry, M.J., Fowler, F.J., Mulley, A.G., Henderson, J.V. and Wennberg, J.E. (1995) Patient reactions to a programme designed to facilitate patient participation in decisions for benign prostatic hyperplasia, *Medical Care*, 33: 771–82.

Bateson, G. (1972) *Steps to an Ecology of Mind*. New York: Ballantine Books.

Beach, W.A. (1995) Preserving and constraining options: 'okays' and 'official' priorities in medical interviews, in G.H. Morris and R.J. Chenail (eds) *The Talk of the Clinic: Explorations in the Analysis of Medical and Therapeutic Discourse*. New Jersey: Lawrence Erlbaum Associates.

Beck, U. (1992) *Risk Society: Towards a New Modernity*. London: Sage.

BMA Board of Medical Education (2004) *Communication Skills Education for Doctors: An Update*. London: British Medical Association.

Boericke, W., Boericke, O. and Savage R. B. (eds) (1990) *Homoeopathic Materia Medica with Repertory*. London: Homoeopathic Book Service.

Bond, S. (1983) Nurses' communication with cancer patients, in J. Wilson-Barnett (ed.) *Nursing Research: Ten Studies in Patient Care*. Chichester: John Wiley and Sons, Ltd.

Botting, D.A. and Cook, R. (2000) Complementary medicine: knowledge, use and attitudes of doctors, *Complementary Therapies in Nursing and Midwifery*, 6: 41–7.

Boyd, E. and Heritage, J. (2006) Taking the history: questioning during comprehensive history taking, in J. Heritage and D.W. Maynard (eds) *Communication in Medical Care: Interaction between Primary Care Physicians and Patients*. Cambridge: Cambridge University Press.

Bradbury, E.T., Kay, S.P.J., Tighe, K.C. and Hewison, J. (1994) Decision making by parents and children in paediatric hand surgery, *British Journal of Plastic Surgery*, 47: 324–30.

Branch Jr, W.T., Kern, D., Haidet, P. et al. (2001) Teaching the human dimensions of care in clinical settings, *Journal of the American Medical Association*, 286: 1067–74.

Britten, N. (2003) Commentary: clinicians' and patients' roles in patient involvement, *Quality and Safety in Health Care*, 12: 87.

Britten, N., Stevenson, F.A., Barry, C.A., Barber, N. and Bradley, C.P. (2000) Misunderstandings in prescribing decisions in general practice: a qualitative study, *British Medical Journal*, 320: 484–8.

Britten, N., Stevenson, F., Gafaranga, J., Barry, C. and Bradley, C. (2004) The expression of aversion to medicines in general practice consultations, *Social Science and Medicine*, 59: 1495–503.

Bugge, C., Entwistle, V. and Watt, I. (2006) The significance for decision-making of information that is not exchanged by patients and health professionals during consultations, *Social Science and Medicine*, 63: 2065–78.

Button, G. (1991) Conversation-in-a-series, in D. Boden and D.H. Zimmerman (eds) *Talk and Social Structure*. Cambridge: Polity Press.

Byrne, G. and Heyman, R. (1997) Understanding nurses' communication with patients in accident and emergency departments using a symbolic interactionist perspective, *Journal of Advanced Nursing*, 26: 93–100.

Byrne, P.S. and Long, B.E.L. (1976) *Doctors Talking to Patients: A Study of the Verbal Behaviours of Doctors in the Consultation*. London: HMSO.

Cahill, J. (1996) Patient participation: a concept analysis, *Journal of Advanced Nursing*, 24(3): 561–71.

Calnan, M. and Gabe, J. (2001) From consumerism to partnership? Britain's National Health Service at the turn of the century, *International Journal of Health Services*, 31(1): 119–31.

Campion, P., Foulkes, J., Neighbour, R. and Tate, P. (2002) Patient-centredness in the MRCGP video examination: analysis of large cohort, *British Medical Journal*, 325: 691–2.

Caris-Verhallen, W., Kerktra, A. and Bensing, J. (1997) The role of communication in nursing care for elderly people: a review of the literature, *Journal of Advanced Nursing*, 25: 915–33.

Cegala, D. J., Mcure, L., Marinelli, T.M. and Post, D.M. (2000) The effects of communication skills training on patients' participation during medical interviews, *Patient Education and Counselling*, 41: 209–22.

Chapman, V. (1983) Planning the nursing care of the patient, in S. Collins and E. Parker (eds) *An Introduction to Nursing*. London: Macmillan Press.

Chappell, P. (1999) *Emotional Healing with Homoeopathy: A Practical Guide*. Dorset: Element.

Chappell, P. and Andrews, D. (1996) *Healing with Homoeopathy*. Dublin: Gill and Macmillan.

Charles, C. and DeMaio, S. (1993) Lay participation in health care decision making: a conceptual framework, *Journal of Health Politics, Policy and Law*, 18(4): 881–904.

Charles, C., Gafni, A. and Whelan, T. (1997) Shared decision-making in the medical encounter: what does it mean? (or it takes at least two to tango), *Social Science and Medicine*, 44(5): 681–92.

Charles, C., Gafni, A. and Whelan, T. (1999) Decision-making in the patient–physician encounter: revisiting the shared treatment decision-making model, *Social Science and Medicine*, 49: 651–61.

Charles-Jones, H., Latimer, J. and May, C. (2003) Transforming general practice: the redistribution of medical work in primary care, *Sociology of Health and Illness*, 25(1): 71–92.

Chatwin, J. and Collins, S. (2002) Communication in the homoeopathic consultation, *The Homoeopath*, 84(Winter): 24–6.

Collins, S. (2005a) Explanations in consultations: the combined effectiveness of doctors' and nurses' communication with patients, *Medical Education*, 39: 785–96.

Collins, S. (2005b) Communicating for a clinical purpose: strategy in interaction in healthcare consultations, *Communication and Medicine*, 2(2): 111–22.

Collins, S., Drew, P., Watt, I. and Entwistle, V. (2005) 'Unilateral' and 'bilateral' practitioner approaches in decision-making about treatment, *Social Science and Medicine*, 61(12): 611–27.

Collins, S., Watt, I., Drew, P., Local, J. and Cullum, N. (2003) *Effective Consultations with Patients: A Comparative Multidisciplinary Study*: *Full report*. London: Economic and Social Research Council.

Cornwall, A. (1996) Towards participatory practice: participatory rural appraisal (PRA) and the participatory process, in K. de Koning and M. Martin (eds) *Participatory Research in Health*. London: Zed Books.

Coulehan, J.L., Platt, F.W., Egener, B. et al. (2001) 'Let me see if I have this right . . .': words that help build empathy. *Annals of Internal Medicine*, 135(3): 221–7.

Coulter, A. (1991) Evaluating the outcomes of health care, in J. Gabe, M. Calnan and M. Bury (eds) *The Sociology of the Health Service*. London: Routledge.

Coulter, A. (1997) Partnerships with patients: the pros and cons of shared clinical decision making, *Journal of Health Services Research and Policy*, 2(2): 112–21.

Coulter, A. (1999) Paternalism or partnership, *British Medical Journal*, 319: 719–20.

Coulter, A. (2002) *The Autonomous Patient: Ending Paternalism in Medical Care*. London: The Stationery Office/Nuffield Trust.

Coulter, A. and Fitzpatrick, R. (2000) The patient's perspective regarding appropriate health care, in G.L. Albrecht, R. Fitzpatrick and R.C. Scrimshaw (eds) *The Handbook of Social Studies in Health and Medicine*. London: Sage.

Coulter, A. and Magee, H. (eds) (2003) *The European Patient of the Future*. Maidenhead: Open University Press.

Coupland, J., Coupland, N. and Robinson, J.D. (1992) 'How are you?': negotiating phatic communion, *Language in Society*, 21: 207–30.

Davidson, J. (1984) Subsequent version of invitations, offers, requests, and proposals dealing with potential or actual rejection, in J.M. Atkinson and J. Heritage, *Studies in Conversation Analysis*. Cambridge: Cambridge University Press.

Davis, A. (ed.) (1978) *Relationships between Doctors and Patients*. Hants: Teakfield Ltd.

Denning, M.L. and Draper, J. (2004) *A Guide to the Consultation Skills Training Videotape*. Made for the Eastern Deanery Postgraduate General Practice Education. www.easterngp.co.uk (accessed 31 October 2006).

Denzin, N.K. (1970) *The Research Act in Sociology: A Theoretical Introduction to Sociological Methods*. London: Butterworths.

Department of Health (1989) *Working for Patients*. London: HMSO.

Department of Health (1992) *The Patient's Charter*. London: HMSO.

Department of Health (1997) *The New NHS: Modern, Dependable*. London: The Stationery Office.

Department of Health (1998) *A First Class Service*. London: The Stationery Office.

Department of Health (1999) *Patient and Public Involvement in the New NHS*. London: The Stationery Office.

Department of Health (2000) *The NHS Plan: A Plan for Investment, a Plan for Reform*. London: The Stationery Office.

Department of Health (2001) *The Expert Patient: A New Approach to Chronic Disease Management for the 21st Century*. London: The Stationery Office.

Department of Health (2003) *Building on the Best: Choice, Responsiveness and Equity in the NHS*. London: The Stationery Office.

Dickinson, D., Wilkie, P. and Harris, M. (1999) Taking medicine: concordance is not compliance, *British Medical Journal*, 319: 787.

Drew, P. (2001) Spotlight on the patient, *TEXT*, 21:(1/2) 261–9.

Drew, P. (2003) Comparative analysis of talk-in-interaction in different institutional settings: a sketch, in P. Glenn, C.D. LeBaron and J. Mandelbaum (eds) *Studies in Language and Social Interaction: In Honor of Robert Hopper*. Mahwah, NJ: Lawrence Erlbaum.

Drew, P., Chatwin, J. and Collins, S. (2001) Conversation analysis: a method for research in health care professional–patient interaction, *Health Expectations*, 4/1: 58–71.

Drew, P. and Heritage, J. (1992) Analyzing talk at work: an introduction, in Drew, P. and Heritage, J., *Talk at Work: Interaction in Institutional Settings*. Cambridge: Cambridge University Press.

Dunn, N. (2002) Commentary: patient centred care: timely, but is it practical?, *British Medical Journal*, 324: 651.

Eastwood, H. (2000) Why are Australian GPs using alternative medicine? Postmodernisation, consumerism and the shift towards holistic health, *Journal of Sociology*, 36: 133–5.

Elwyn, G., Edwards, A. and Kinnersley, P. (1999) Shared decision-making in primary care: the neglected second half of the consultation, *British Journal of General Practice*, 49: 477–82.

Elwyn, G., Edwards, A., Kinnersley, P. and Grol, R. (2000) Shared decision-making and the concept of equipoise: the competencies of involving patients in healthcare choices, *British Journal of General Practice*, 50(460): 892–7.

Elwyn, G., Edwards, A., Mowle, S. et al. (2001) Measuring the involvement of patients in shared decision-making: a systematic review of instruments, *Patient Education and Counselling*, 43: 5–22.

Elwyn, G., Edwards, A. and Rhydderch, M. (2003a) Shared decision-making in clinical practice, in R. Jones, N. Britten, L. Culpepper et al. (eds) *Oxford Textbook of Primary Medical Care*. Oxford: Oxford University Press.

Elwyn, G., Edwards, A., Wensing, M. et al. (2003b) Shared decision making: developing the OPTION scale for measuring patient involvement, *Quality and Safety in Health Care*, 12: 93–9.

Elwyn, G. and Gwyn, R. (1999) Narrative based medicine: stories we hear and stories we tell: analysing talk in clinical practice, *British Medical Journal*, 318: 186–8.

Elwyn, G., Hutchings, H., Edwards, A. et al. (2005) The OPTION scale: measuring the extent that clinicians involve patients in decision-making tasks, *Health Expectations*, 8(1): 34–42.

Emanuel, E.J. and Emanuel, L.L. (1997) Preserving community in health care, *Journal of Health Politics, Policy and Law*, 22(1): 147–84.

Entwistle, V.A., Sowden, J.A. and Watt, I.S. (1998) Evaluating interventions to promote patient involvement in decision-making: by what criteria should effectiveness be judged? *Journal of Health Service Research Policy*, 3(2): 100–7.

Entwistle, V.A. and Watt, I.S. (2006) Patient involvement in treatment decision-making: the case for a broader conceptual framework, *Patient Education and Counselling*, 63: 268–78.

Entwistle, V., Watt, I., Gilhooly, K. et al. (2004) Assessing patients' participation and quality of decision-making: insights from a study of routine practice in diverse settings, *Patient Education and Counselling*, 55: 105–13.

Eysenbach, G. (2000) Towards ethical guidelines for dealing with unsolicited patient emails and giving teleadvice in the absence of a pre-existing patient–physician relationship – systematic review and expert survey, *Journal of Medical Internet Research*, 2(1), e1. http://www.jmir.org/2000/1/e1/index.htm (accessed 30 August 2004).

Fallowfield, L.J., Jenkins, V.A. and Beveridge, H.A. (2002) Truth may hurt but deceit hurts more: communication in palliative care, *Palliative Medicine*, 16: 297–303.

Farrell, C. (2004) *Patient and Public Involvement in Health: The Evidence for Policy Implementation. A Summary of the Results of the Health in Partnership Research Programme*. London: Department of Health.

Feingold, E. (1977) Citizen participation: a review of the issues, in H.M. Rosen, J.M. Metsch and S. Levey, *The Consumer and the Health Care System: Social and Managerial Perspectives*. New York: Spectrum.

Firth, A. (1995) Talking for change: commodity negotiating by telephone, in A. Firth (ed.) *The Discourse of Negotiation: Studies of Language in the Workplace*. Oxford: Pergamon Press, pp. 183–222.

Fitzgerald, M. (2002) Meeting the needs of individuals, in J. Daly, S. Speedy, D. Jackson and P. Darbyshire (eds) *Contexts of Nursing: An Introduction*. Oxford: Blackwell Publishing.

Ford, S., Schofield, T. and Hope, T. (2006) Observing decision-making in the general practice consultation: who makes which decisions? *Health Expectations*, 9(2): 130–7.

Foss, C. and Ellefsen, B. (2002) The value of combining qualitative and quantitative approaches in nursing research by means of a method triangulation, *Journal of Advanced Nursing*, 40: 242–8.

Foster, N.E., Thompson, K.A., Baxter, G.D. and Allen, J.M. (1999) Management of nonspecific low back pain by physiotherapists in Britain and Ireland, *Spine*, 24: 1332–42.

Frankel, R.M. and West, C. (1991) Miscommunication in medicine, in N. Coupland, H. Giles and J.M. Wiemann (eds) *'Miscommunication' and Problematic Talk*. London: Sage.

Gabe, J., Olumide, G. and Bury, M. (2004) 'It takes three to tango': a framework for understanding patient partnership in paediatric clinics, *Social Science and Medicine*, 59: 1071–9.

Gafaranga, J. and Britten, N. (2003) 'Fire away': the opening sequence in general practice consultations, *Family Practice*, 20: 242–7.

Gafaranga, J. and Britten, N. (2004) Formulation in general practice consultations, *TEXT*, 24: 147–70.

Gafaranga, J. and Britten, N. (2005) Talking an institution into being: the opening sequence in general practice consultations, in K. Richards and P. Seedhouse (eds) *Applying Conversation Analysis*. New York: Palgrave Macmillan.

Garfinkel, H. (1967) *Studies in Ethnomethodology*. Englewood Cliffs, NJ: Prentice Hall.

General Medical Council (2001) *Good Medical Practice*. London: General Medical Council.

Gilhooly, K. and Green, C. (1996) Protocol analysis: theoretical background, in J.T.E. Richardson (ed.) *Handbook of Qualitative Research Methods for Psychology and the Social Sciences*. Leicester: British Psychological Society, pp. 43–54.

Gill, V.T. and Maynard, D.W. (2006) Explaining illness: patients' proposals and physicians' responses, in J. Heritage and D.W. Maynard (eds) *Communication in Medical Care: Interaction between Primary Care Physicians and Patients*. Cambridge: Cambridge University Press.

Glasgow Homoeopathic Hospital (2006) *Creating Healing Spaces*. www.adhom.org.uk (accessed 30 October 2006).

Glenister, D. (1994) Patient participation in psychiatric services: a literature review and proposal for a research strategy, *Journal of Advanced Nursing*, 19(4): 802–11.

Graumann, C.F. (1995) Commonality, mutuality, reciprocity: a conceptual introduction, in I. Marková, C.F. Graumann and K. Foppa (eds) *Mutualities in Dialogue*. Cambridge: Cambridge University Press.

Green, C. and Gilhooly, K. (1996) Protocol analysis: practical implementation, in J.T.E. Richardson (ed.) *Handbook of Qualitative Research Methods for Psychology and the Social Sciences*. Leicester: British Psychological Society, pp. 55–74.

Greenfield, S., Kaplan, S. and Ware, J.E. Jr. (1985) Expanding patient involvement in care: effects on patient outcomes, *Annals of Internal Medicine*, 102: 520–8.

Greenfield, S., Kaplan, S.H. and Ware, J.E. Jr. (1988) Patients' participation in medical care: effects on blood sugar and quality of life in diabetes, *Journal of General Internal Medicine*, 3: 448–57.

Greenhalgh, T. and Hurwitz, B. (1999) Why study narrative?, *British Medical Journal*, 318: 48–50.

Greenson, R.R. (1967) *The Technique and Practice of Psychoanalysis*. Madison, WI: International Universities Press.

Guadagnoli, E. and Ward, P. (1998) Patient participation in decision-making, *Social Science and Medicine*, 47(3): 329–39.

Guba, E.G. and Lincoln, Y.S. (1994) *Competing Paradigms in Qualitative Research*. London: Sage.

Gumperz, J. (1982) *Discourse Strategies*. Cambridge: Cambridge University Press.

Gwyn, R. (2002) *Communicating Health and Illness*. London: Sage.

Hall J.A., Horgan, T.G., Stein, T.S. and Roter, D.L. (2002) Liking in the physician–patient relationship, *Patient Education and Counselling*, 48(1): 69–77.

Hall, J.A., Roter, D.L. and Katz, N.R. (1988) Meta-analysis of correlates of provider behaviour in medical encounters, *Medical Care*, 26: 657–75.

Hartrick, G. (1997) Relational capacity: the foundation for interpersonal nursing practice, *Journal of Advanced Nursing*, 26(3): 523.

Hasman, A., Coulter, A. and Askham, J. (2006) *Education for Partnership: Developments in Medical Education*. Oxford: Picker Institute Europe.

Haywood, K., Marshall, S. and Fitzpatrick, R. (2006) Patient participation in the consultation process: a structured review of intervention strategies, *Patient Education and Counselling*, 63: 12–23.

Heath, C. (1992) The delivery and reception of diagnosis in the general practice consultation, in P. Drew and J. Heritage (eds) *Talk at Work: Interaction in Institutional Settings*. Cambridge: Cambridge University Press.

Heritage, J. and Maynard, D.W. (eds) (2006) *Communication in Medical Care: Interaction between Primary Care Physicians and Patients*. Cambridge: Cambridge University Press.

Heritage, J. and Robinson, J.D. (2006) Accounting for the visit: giving reasons for seeking medical care, in J. Heritage and D.W. Maynard (eds) *Communication in Medical Care: Interaction between Primary Care Physicians and Patients*. Cambridge: Cambridge University Press.

Heritage, J. and Stivers, T. (1999) Online commentary in acute medical visits: a method of shaping patient expectations, *Social Science and Medicine*, 49: 1501–17.

Heritage, J. and Watson, R. (1979) Formulations as conversational objects, in G. Psathas (ed.) *Everyday Language: Studies in Ethnomethodology*. New York: Irvington.

Hirschman, A. (1970) *Exit, Voice and Loyalty*. Cambridge, MA: Harvard University Press.

Hogg, C. (1999) *Patients, Power and Politics: From Patients to Citizens*. London: Sage.

Hoggett, P. (2001) Agency, rationality and social policy, *Journal of Social Policy*, 30(1): 37–56.

Holman, H. and Lorig, K. (2000) Patients as partners in managing chronic disease, *British Medical Journal*, 320: 526–7.

House of Lords (2000) *Complementary and Alternative Medicine*. London: Stationery Office.

Houtkoop, H. (1986) Summarizing in doctor–patient interaction, in T. Ensink, A. Van Essen and T. Van Geest (eds) *Discourse and Public Life*. Dordrecht/ Providence, RI: Foris Publications.

Howie, J.G.R., Heaney, D. and Maxwell, M. (2004) Quality, core values and general practice consultation: issues of definition, measurement and delivery, *Family Practice*, 21: 458–68.

Hunt, M. (1991) Being friendly and informal: reflected in nurses', terminally ill patients' and relatives' conversations at home, *Journal of Advanced Nursing*, 16: 929–38.

Hunter, D. (2004) A structural perspective on health care reform, *Journal of Health Services Research and Policy*, 9(1): 51–3.

Hunter, K.M. (1991) *Doctors' Stories: The Narrative Structure of Medical Knowledge*. Princeton, NJ: Princeton University Press.

Jarrett, N. and Payne, S. (1995) A selective review of the literature on nurse–patient communication: has the patient's contribution been neglected? *Journal of Advanced Nursing*, 22: 72–8.

Jefferson, G. (1984) Transcript notation, in J.M. Atkinson and J. Heritage (eds) *Structures of Social Action: studies in conversation analysis*. Cambridge: Cambridge University Press.

Jefferson, G. (1985) An exercise in the transcription and analysis of laughter, in T. Van Dijk (ed.) *Handbook of Discourse Analysis*, vol. 3. London: Academia Press.

Jefferson, G. (1990) List construction as a task and a resource, in G. Psathas (ed.) *Interactional Competence*. Washington, DC: University Press of America, pp. 63–92.

Jones, A. (2003) Nurses talking to patients: exploring conversation analysis as a means of researching nurse/patient communication, *International Journal of Nursing Studies*, 40(6): 609–18.

Jones, A. (2005) 'I've just got to ask you some questions': an exploration of how nurses and patients accomplish initial assessments in hospitals, unpublished PhD thesis, Swansea University.

Jones, I.R., Berney, L., Kelly, M. et al. (2004) Is patient involvement possible when decisions involve scarce resources? A qualitative study of decision-making in primary care, *Social Science and Medicine*, 59(1): 93–102.

Jones, R., Britten, N., Culpepper, L. et al. (eds) (2003) *Oxford Textbook of Primary Medical Care*. Oxford: Oxford University Press.

Jump, J., Yarbrough, L., Kilpatrick, S. and Cable, T. (1998) Physicians' attitudes toward complementary and alternative medicine, *Integrative Medicine*, 1(4): 149–53.

Kacperek, L. (1997) Non-verbal communication: the importance of listening, *British Journal of Nursing*, 6(5): 275–9.

Kings Fund (2006) *Improving the Patient Experience – Celebrating Achievement: Enhancing the Healing Environment Programme*. Norwich: The Stationery Office.

Kitzinger, J. and Barbour, R.S. (1999) Introduction: the challenge and promise of focus groups, in R.S. Barbour and J. Kitzinger (eds) *Developing Focus Group Research*. London: Sage.

Kraetschmer, N., Sharpe, N., Urowitz, S. and Deber, R.B. (2004) How does trust affect patient preferences for participation in decision-making? *Health Expectations, 7*: 317–26.

Kurtz, S., Silverman, J. and Draper, J. (1998) *Teaching and Learning Communication Skills in Medicine*. Oxford: Radcliffe Medical Press.

Lask, B. (2002) Daily regimen and compliance with treatment: concordance respects beliefs and wishes of patients, *British Medical Journal*, 324: 425.

Latimer, J. (2000) *The Conduct of Care*. Oxford: Blackwell Science.

Launer, J. (1999) A narrative approach to mental health in general practice, *British Medical Journal*, 318: 117–19.

Le May, A., Mulhall, A. and Alexander, C. (1998) Bridging the research-practice gap: exploring the research cultures of practitioners and managers, *Journal of Advanced Nursing*, 28(2): 428–37.

Lindfors, P. (2005) *Homeopaatin vastaanotolla – tutkimus vuorovaikutuksesta ja päätöksenteossa*. [On Homoepathic Encounter: a Study of Interaction and Decision-Making Practices]. Acta Electronica Universitatis Tamperensis, 456. Tampere: Tampere University Press.

Lindfors, P. and Raevaara, L. (2005) Discussing patient's drinking and eating habits in medical and homoeopathic consultations, *Communication and Medicine*, 2(2): 137–49.

Little, P., Everitt, H., Williamson, I. et al. (2001) Preferences of patients for patient centred approach to consultation in primary care: observational study, *British Medical Journal*, 322: 1–7.

Lupton, C., Peckham, S. and Taylor, P. (1998) *Managing Public Involvement in Healthcare Purchasing*. Buckingham: Open University Press.

Macloed Clark, J. (1983) Nurse–patient communication – an analysis of conversations from surgical wards, in J. Wilson-Barnett (ed.) *Nursing Research: Ten Studies in Patient Care*. Chichester: John Wiley and Sons, Ltd.

Makoul, G., Arntson, P. and Schofield, T. (1995) Health promotion in primary care: physician–patient communication and decision making about prescription medications, *Social Science and Medicine*, 41: 1241–54.

May, C., Allison, G., Chapple, A. et al. (2004) Framing the doctor–patient relationship in chronic illness: a comparative study of general practitioners' accounts, *Sociology of Health and Illness*, 26: 135–58.

Maynard, D.W. (1992) On clinicians co-implicating recipients' perspective in the delivery of diagnostic news, in P. Drew and J. Heritage (eds) *Talk at Work: Interaction in Institutional Settings*. Cambridge: Cambridge University Press.

Mays, N. and Pope, C. (2000) Assessing quality in qualitative research, *British Medical Journal*, 320: 50–2.

McEwan, J., Martini, C.J.M. and Wilkins, N. (1983) *Participation in Health*. London: Croom Helm.

McKinstry, B. (2000) Do patients wish to be involved in decision making in the consultation? A cross-sectional survey with video vignettes, *British Medical Journal*, 321: 867–71.

McWhinney, I.R. (1972) Beyond diagnosis: an approach to the integration of behavioural science and clinical medicine, *New England Journal of Medicine*, 287: 384–7.

Mercer, S.W. and Howie, J.G. (2006) CQI-2 – a new measure of holistic interpersonal care in primary care consultations, *British Journal of General Practice*, 56(525): 262–8.

Mercer, S.W., Maxwell, M., Heaney, D. and Watt, G.C. (2004) The consultation and relational empathy (CARE) measure: development and preliminary validation and reliability of an empathy-based consultation process measure, *Family Practice*, 21(6): 699–705.

Mercer, S.W. and Reilly, D. (2004) A qualitative study of patients' views on the consultation at the Glasgow Homoeopathic Hospital, an NHS integrative complementary and orthodox medical care unit, *Patient Education and Counselling*, 53(1): 13–18.

Mercer, S.W., Reilly, D. and Watt, G.C.M. (2002) The importance of empathy in the enablement of patients attending the Glasgow Homoeopathic Hospital, *British Journal of General Practice*, 52: 901–5.

Mercer, S.W. and Reynolds, W. (2002) Empathy and quality of care, *British Journal of General Practice*, 52 (Suppl): S9–S12.

Middleton, J.F., McKinley, R.K. and Gillies, C.L. (2006) Effect of patient completed agenda forms and doctors' education about the agenda on the outcome of consultations: randomised controlled trial, *British Medical Journal*, 332: 1238–41.

Miller, J. and Glassner, B. (2004) The 'inside' and the 'outside': finding realities in interviews, in D. Silverman (ed.) *Qualitative Research: Theory, Method and Practice*, 2nd edn. London: Sage.

Mishler, E.G. (1984) *The Discourse of Medicine: Dialectics of Medical Interviews*. Norwood, NJ: Ablex.

Morgan, D.L. (1997) *Focus Groups as Qualitative Research*, 2nd edn. London: Sage.

Mullen, P. and Spurgeon, P. (2000) *Priority Setting and the Public*. Abingdon: Radcliff Medical Press.

National Assembly for Wales (2001) *Improving Health in Wales: A Plan for the NHS with its Partners*. Cardiff: National Assembly for Wales.

NHS Executive (1996) *Patient Partnership: Building a Collaborative Strategy*. Leeds: NHS Executive.

Nolan, M. and Caddock, K. (1996) Assessment: identifying the barriers to good practice, *Health and Social Care in the Community*, 4(2): 77–85.

Nolan, M., Grant, G. and Nolan, J. (1995) Busy doing nothing: activity and interaction levels amongst differing populations of elderly patients, *Journal of Advanced Nursing*, 2: 528–38.

Olszewski, D. and Jones, L. (1998) *Putting People in the Picture: Information for Patients and the Public about Illness and Treatment. A Review of the Literature*. Edinburgh: Scottish Association of Health Councils/Scottish Health Feedback.

Paley, J. (2001) An archaeology of caring knowledge, *Journal of Advanced Nursing*, 36(2): 188–98.

Parahoo, K. (1997) *Nursing Research: Principles, Process and Issues*. Basingstoke: Palgrave.

Parahoo, K. (2000) A comparison of pre-Project 2000 and Project 2000 nurses' perceptions of their research training, research needs and of their use of research in clinical areas, *Journal of Advanced Nursing*, 29(1): 237–45.

Parsons, T. (1951) *The Social System*. Glencoe, IL: The Free Press.

Peräkylä, A. (1995) *Aids Counselling: Institutional Interaction and Clinical Practice*. Cambridge: Cambridge University Press.

Peräkylä, A. (1997) Conversation analysis: a new model of research in doctor–patient communication, *Journal of the Royal Society of Medicine*, 90: 205–8.

Peräkylä, A. (1998) Authority and accountability: the delivery of diagnosis in primary health care, *Social Psychology Quarterly*, 61: 310–20.

Peräkylä, A. (2002) Agency and authority: extended responses to diagnostic statements in primary care encounters, *Research on Language and Social Interaction*, 35(2): 219–47.

Peräkylä, A. (2006) Patients' responses to interpretations: a dialogue between conversation analysis and psychoanalytic theory, *Communication & Medicine*, 2(2): 163–76.

Peräkylä, A., Ruusuvuori, J. and Vehviläinen, S. (2005) Introduction: professional theories and institutional interaction, *Communication & Medicine*, 2(2): 105–10.

Peräkylä, A. and Vehviläinen, S. (2003) Conversation analysis and the professional stocks of interactional knowledge, *Discourse and Society*, 14(6): 727–50.

Pfeffer, N. and Coote, A. (1991) *Is Quality Good for You?* Social Policy Paper No. 5. London: Institute for Public Policy Research.

Pomerantz, A. (1984) Agreeing and disagreeing with assessments: some features of preferred/dispreferred turn-shapes, in J.M. Atkinson and J. Heritage (eds) *Structures of Social Action: Studies in Conversation Analysis*. Cambridge: Cambridge University Press.

Pomerantz, A., Fehr, B.J. and Ende, J. (1997) When supervising physicians see patients: strategies used in difficult situations, *Human Communication Research*, 23: 589–615.

Pope, C. and Mays, N. (eds) (2006) *Qualitative Research in Health Care*, 3rd edn. London: BMJ Books.

Razum, O. and Gerhardus, A. (1999) Methodological triangulation in public health research – advancement or mirage? *Tropical Medicine and International Health*, 4: 243–4.

Reilly, D. (2001) Enhancing human healing, *British Medical Journal*, 322: 120–1.

Reynolds, W. (2000) *The Measurement and Development of Empathy in Nursing*. Aldershot: Ashgate Publishing Ltd.

Richards, K. (2005) Introduction, in K. Richards and P. Seedhouse (eds) *Applying Conversation Analysis*. New York: Palgrave Macmillan.

Richards, T. (1990) Chasms in communication, *British Medical Journal*, 301: 1407–8.

Richards, T. (1998) Partnership with patients. *British Medical Journal*, 316: 85–6.

Rifkin, S.B. and Pridmore, P. (2001) *Partners in Planning: Information, Participation and Empowerment*. London: Macmillan.

Ring, A., Dowrick, C., Humphris, G. and Salmon, P. (2004) Do patients with unexplained symptoms pressurise general practitioners for somatic treatment? A qualitative study, *British Medical Journal*, 328: 1057–62.

Robinson, J. (2003) An interactional structure of medical activities during acute visits and its implications for patients' participation, *Health Communication*, 15(1): 27–59.

Robinson, J. (2006) Soliciting patients' presenting concerns, in J. Heritage and D.W. Maynard (eds) *Communication in Medical Care: Interaction between Primary Care Physicians and Patients*. Cambridge: Cambridge University Press.

Rogers, B.L. (1989) Concepts, analysis and the development of nursing knowledge: the evolutionary cycle, *Journal of Advanced Nursing*, 14(4): 330–5.

Roper, N., Logan, W. and Tierney, A. (1996) *The Elements of Nursing: A Model for Nursing. Based on a Model of Living*, 4th edn. London: Churchill Livingstone.

Rost, K., Carter, W. and Inui, T. (1989) Introduction of information during the initial medical visit: consequences for patient follow-through with physician recommendations for medication, *Social Science and Medicine*, 28(4): 315–21.

Roter, D.L. (1977) Patient participation in the patient–provider interaction: the effects of patient question asking on the quality of the interaction, satisfaction, and compliance, *Health Education Monographs*, 5: 281–315.

Roter, D.L. (2000) The enduring and evolving nature of the patient–physician relationship, *Patient Education and Counselling*, 39: 5–15.

Roter, D.L. and Hall, J.A. (1992) *Doctors Talking with Patients, Patients Talking with Doctors: Improving Communication in Medical Visits*. Westport, CT: Auburn House.

Roter, D.L. and Larson, S. (2002) The Roter interaction analysis system (RIAS): utility and flexibility for analysis of medical interactions, *Patient Education and Counselling*, 46(4): 243–51.

Rudebeck, C.E. (2002) Imagination and empathy in the consultation, *British Journal of General Practice*, 52: 450–3.

Ruusuvuori, J. (2000) Control in the medical consultation: giving and receiving the reason for the visit in Finnish primary care encounters, Acta Universitatis Tamperensis, 16. http://acta.fi./pdf/951–44–4755–7.pdf

Ruusuvuori, J. (2005) Comparing homoeopathic and general practice consultations: the case of problem presentation, *Communication & Medicine*, 2(2): 123–36.

Rycroft, C. (1995) *A Critical Dictionary of Psychoanalysis*. London: Penguin.

Sacks, H., Schegloff, E. and Jefferson, G. (1974) A simple systematics for the organization of turn taking during conversations, in J. Schenken (ed.) *Studies in the Organization of Conversational Interaction*. New York: Academic Press.

Scambler, G. and Britten, N. (2001) System, lifeworld and doctor–patient interaction, in G. Scambler (ed.) *Habermas, Critical Theory and Health*. London: Routledge.

Schegloff, E. (1992) On talk and its institutional occasions, in P. Drew and J. Heritage (eds) *Talk at Work: Interaction in Institutional Settings*. London: Sage.

Schofield, P.E., Butow, P.N., Thompson, J.F., Tattersall, M.H.N., Beeney, L.J. and Dunn, S.M. (2003) Psychological responses of patients receiving a diagnosis of cancer, *Annals of Oncology*, 14(1): 48–56.

Scottish Executive Health Department (2000) *Our Naional Health: A Plan for Action, a Plan for Change*. Edinburgh: The Stationery Office.

Scottish Executive Health Department (2003) *Partnership for Care*. Edinburgh: The Stationery Office.

Searle, J.R. (1969) *Speech Acts*. Cambridge: Cambridge University Press.

Sefi, S. (1988) Health visitors talking to mothers, *Health Visitor* 61(1): 7–10.

Shih, F.J. (1998) Triangulation in nursing research: issues of conceptual clarity and purpose, *Journal of Advanced Nursing*, 28: 631–41.

Silverman, D. (1987) *Communication and Medical Practice: Social Relations and the Clinic*. Bristol: Sage.

Silverman, D. (1993) *Interpreting Qualitative Data: Methods for Analysing Talk, Text and Interaction*. London: Sage.

Sim, J. and Sharp, K. (1998) A critical appraisal of the role of triangulation in nursing research, *International Journal of Nursing Studies*, 35: 23–31.

Slater, N. (2000) *Appetite*. London: Fourth Estate.

Sorjonen, M-L. (2001) *Responding in Conversation: A Study of Response Particles in Finnish*. Amsterdam: John Benjamins.

Spencer, J. and Dales, J. (2006) Meeting the needs of simulated patients and caring for the person behind them?, *Medical Education*, 40(1): 3–5.

Squier, R. (1990) A model of empathetic understanding and adherence to treatment regimens in practitioner–patient relationships, *Social Science and Medicine*, 55: 669–73.

Stevenson, F.A., Barry, C.A., Britten, N., Barber, N. and Bradley, C.P. (2000) Doctor–patient communication about drugs: the evidence for shared decision making, *Social Science and Medicine*, 50: 829–40.

Stevenson, F.A., Britten, N., Barry, C.A., Bradley, C.P. and Barber, N. (2003) Self treatment and its discussion in medical consultations: how is medical pluralism managed in practice? *Social Science and Medicine*, 57(3): 513–27.

Stewart, M. (1995) Effective physician–patient communication and health outcomes: a review, *Canadian Medical Association Journal*, 152(9): 1423–33.

Stewart, M., Brown, J.B., Weston, W.W. et al. (1995) *Patient-Centred Medicine: Transforming the Clinical Method*. Oxford: Radcliffe Medical Press Ltd.

Stewart, M.A. (2001) Towards a global definition of patient-centred care, *British Medical Journal*, 322: 444–5.

Stivers, T. (2002) Participating in decisions about treatment: overt parent pressure for antibiotic medication in pediatric encounters, *Social Science and Medicine*, 54(7): 1111–30.

Stivers, T. (2005a) Parent resistance to physicians' treatment recommendations: one resource for initiating a negotiation of the treatment decision, *Health Communication*, 18: 41–74.

Stivers, T. (2005b) Non-antibiotic treatment recommendations: delivery formats and implications for parent resistance, *Social Science and Medicine*, 60: 949–64.

Stivers, T. and Heritage, J. (2001) Breaking the sequential mold: 'Answering more than the question' during comprehensive history taking, *TEXT*, 21:(1/2): 151–86.

Street, R.L. (1991) Information-giving in medical consultations: the influence of patients' communicative styles and personal characteristics, *Social Science and Medicine*, 32: 541–8.

Street, R.L. and Millay, B. (2001) Analyzing patient participation in medical encounters, *Health Communication*, 13: 61–73.

Strong, P. (1979) *The Ceremonial Order of the Clinic: Parents, Doctors and Medical Bureaucracies*. London: Routledge and Kegan Paul.

Sullivan, M. (2003) The new subjective medicine: taking the patient's point of view on health care and health, *Social Science and Medicine*, 56(7): 1595–604.

Sully, P. and Dallas, J. (2005) *Essential Communication Skills for Nursing*. Edinburgh: Elsevier Mosby.

Sutherland, H., Llewellyn-Thomas H.A., Lockwood, G.A. et al. (1989) Cancer patients: their desire for information and participation in treatment decisions, *Journal of the Royal Society of Medicine*, 82: 260–3.

Szasz, T.S. and Hollender, M.H. (1956) A contribution to the philosophy of medicine: the basic models of the doctor–patient relationship, *Archives of Internal Medicine*, 97(5): 585–92.

Thomas, K., Carr, J., Westlake, L. and Williams, B. (1991) Use of non-orthodox and conventional health care in Britain, *British Medical Journal*, 302: 207–10.

Thompson, A. (1995) Customizing the public for health care: what's in a label? in I. Kirkpatrick and M. Martinez Lucio (eds) *The Politics of Quality in the Public Sector*. London: Routledge.

Thompson, A.G.H. (1999) New millennium, new values: citizen participation as the democratic ideal in health care, *International Journal for Quality in Health Care*, 11(6): 461–4.

Thompson, A.G.H. (2007). The meaning of patient involvement and participation in health care consultations: a taxonomy. *Social Science and Medicine*. 64: 1297–1310.

Tovey, P. (1997) Contingent legitimacy: UK alternative practitioners and intersectoral acceptance, *Social Science and Medicine*, 45(7): 1129–33.

Tuckett, D., Boulton, M., Olson, C. and Williams, A. (1985) *Meetings Between Experts: An Approach to Sharing Ideas in Medical Consultations*. London: Tavistock Publications.

UK Parliament (2001a) *Learning from Bristol: The Report of the Public Inquiry into Children's Heart Surgery at the Bristol Royal Infirmary 1984–1995*, Cm 5207. London: The Stationery Office.

UK Parliament (2001b) *Health and Social Care Act*. London: The Stationery Office.

UNICEF (2001) *The Participation Rights of Adolescents: A Strategic Approach*, Working Paper PD/05–01. New York: UNICEF.

Vincent, C. and Furnham, A. (1996) Why do patients turn to complementary medicine? An empirical study, *British Journal of Clinical Psychology*, 35: 37–48.

Vithoulkas, G. (1980) *Science of Homoeopathy*. New York: Grove Press.

Walker, E. (1994) Negotiating work, unpublished PhD, University of York.

Wennberg, J.E. (2002) Unwarranted variations in healthcare delivery: implications for academic medical centres, *British Medical Journal*, 325(7370): 961–4.

West, C. (2006) Co-ordinating closings in primary care visits: producing continuity of care, in J. Heritage and D W. Maynard (eds) *Communication in Medical Care: Interaction between Primary Care Physicians and Patients*. Cambridge: Cambridge University Press.

Whelan, T.J., Levine, M.N., Gafni, A. et al. (1995) Breast irradiation postlumpectomy: development and evaluation of a decision instrument, *Journal of Clinical Oncology*, 13: 847–53.

White, D. (2000) Consumer and community participation: a reassessment of process, impact and value, in G. Albrecht, R. Fitzpatrick, and S.C. Scrimshaw (eds) *Handbook of Social Studies in Health and Medicine*. London: Sage.

Whittington, D. and McLaughlin, C. (2000) Finding time for patients: an exploration of nurses' time allocation in an acute psychiatric setting, *Journal of Psychiatric and Mental Health Nursing*, 7: 259–68.

Williams, A. (2000) *Nursing, Medicine and Primary Care*. Buckingham: Open University Press.

Williams, B. and Grant, G. (1998) Defining 'people-centredness': making the implicit explicit, *Health and Social Care in the Community*, 6(2): 84–94.

Winkler, F. (1987) Consumerism in health care – beyond the supermarket model, *Policy and Politics*, 15(1): 1–8.

Wooffitt, R. (2001) Researching psychic practitioners: Conversation Analysis, in

M. Wetherell, S. Taylor and S.J. Yates (eds) *Discourse as Data: A Guide for Analysis*. London: Sage Publications in association with the Open University.

World Health Organization (1978) *Primary Health Care*. Geneva: World Health Organization.

World Health Organization (2005) *Health Promotion in Hospitals: Evidence and Quality Management*. Copenhagen: World Health Organization.

Young, A.S., Klap, R., Sherbourne, C. et al. (2001) The quality of care for depressive and anxiety disorders in the United States, *Archives of General Psychiatry*, 58:55–63.

Index

Page numbers in *italics* refer to figures and tables.

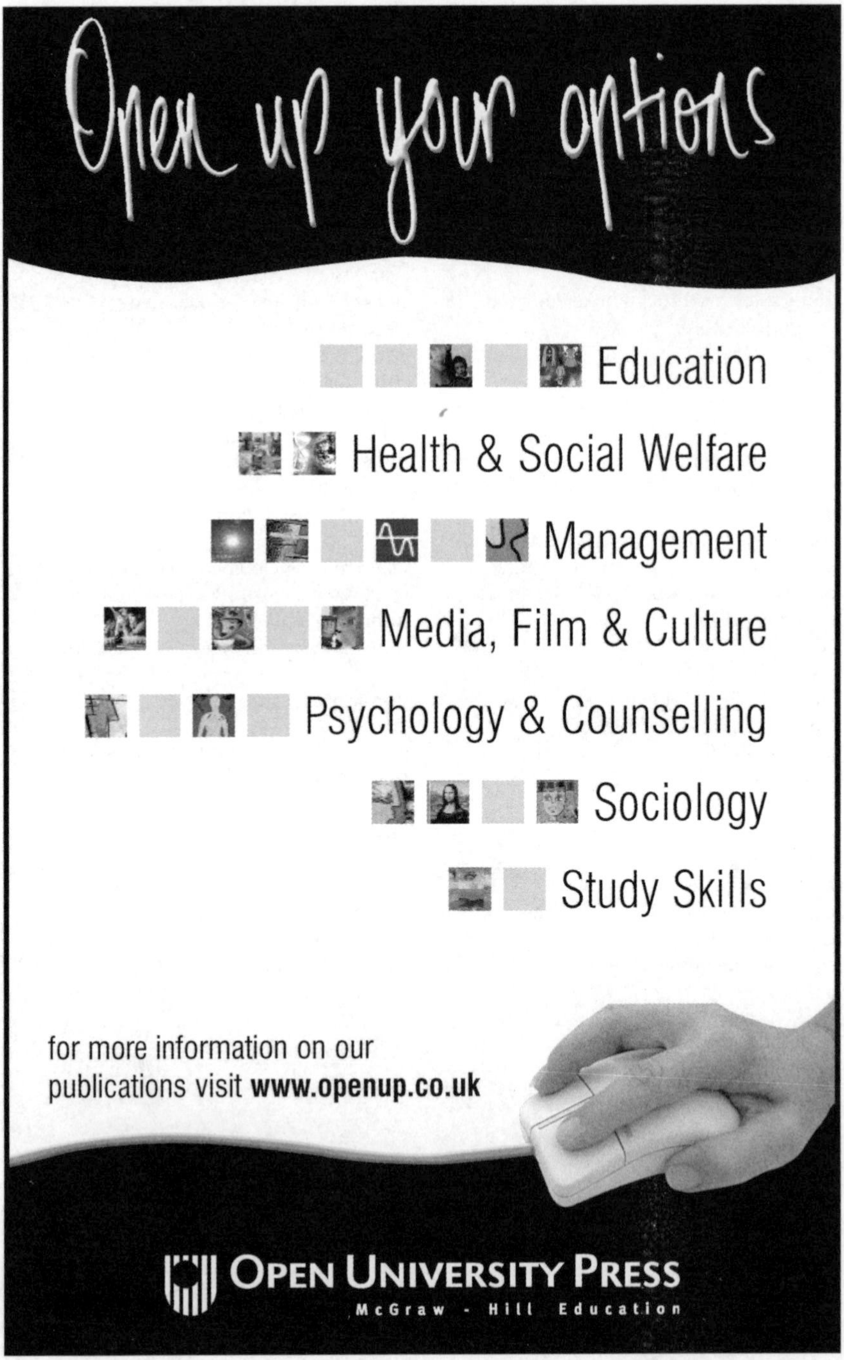
Open up your options
Education
Health & Social Welfare
Management
Media, Film & Culture
Psychology & Counselling
Sociology
Study Skills
for more information on our publications visit www.openup.co.uk
OPEN UNIVERSITY PRESS
McGraw - Hill Education